Healing
and the
Grief Process

Healing and the Grief Process

SALLY S. ROACH, MSN, RN, CNS
Assistant Professor
School of Health Sciences
The University of Texas at Brownsville and
Texas Southmost College

BEATRIZ C. NIETO, MSN, RN, CNS
Assistant Professor
School of Health Sciences
The University of Texas Pan American

Delmar Publishers

An International Thomson Publishing Company

Albany • Bonn • Boston • Cincinnati • Detroit • London
Madrid • Melbourne • Mexico City • New York • Pacific Grove
Paris • San Francisco • Singapore • Tokyo • Toronto • Washington

NOTICE TO THE READER

Cover Design: Spiral Design
Cover Illustration: Kirsten Soderlind

Delmar Staff
Acquisitions Editor: Bill Burgower
Assistant Editor: Hilary A. Schrauf
Senior Project Editor: Judith Boyd Nelson
Production Coordinator: Barbara A. Bullock
Art and Design Coordinator: Carole Keohane

COPYRIGHT © 1997
By Delmar Publishers
a division of International Thomson Publishing Inc.

The ITP logo is a trademark under license.

Printed in the United States of America

For more information, contact:

Delmar Publishers
3 Columbia Circle, Box 15015
Albany, New York 12212-5015

International Thomson Publishing Europe
Berkshire House 168-173
High Holborn
London, WC1V 7AA
England

Thomas Nelson Australia
102 Dodds Street
South Melbourne, 3205
Victoria, Australia

Nelson Canada
1120 Birchmount Road
Scarborough, Ontario
Canada, M1K 5G4

International Thomson Editores
Campos Eliseos 385, Piso 7
Col Polanco
11560 Mexico D F Mexico

International Thomson Publishing GmbH
Konigswinterer Strasse 418
53227 Bonn
Germany

International Thomson Publishing Asia
221 Henderson Road
#05-10 Henderson Building
Singapore 0315

International Thomson Publishing—Japan
Hirakawacho Kyowa Building, 3F
2-2-1 Hirakawacho
Chiyoda-ku, Tokyo 102
Japan

1 2 3 4 5 6 7 8 9 10 XXX 02 01 00 99 98 97 96

Library of Congress Cataloging-in-Publication Data

Roach, Sally S.
   Healing and the grief process / Sally S. Roach, Beatriz C. Nieto.
      p.   cm. — (Nurse as healer series)
   Includes bibliographical references and index.
   ISBN 0-8273-6968-9
    1. Nursing — Psychological aspects.   2. Bereavement — Psychological
aspects.   3. Grief.   4. Loss (Psychology).   I. Nieto, Beatriz C.
II. Title.   III. Series.
RT86.R55   1997
155.9'37'024613 — dc20

96–576
CIP

INTRODUCTION TO NURSE AS HEALER SERIES

LYNN KEEGAN, PhD, RN, FAAN, Series Editor

*Associate Professor, School of Nursing,
University of Texas Health Science Center at San Antonio
and Director of BodyMind Systems, Temple, TX*

To nurse means to care for or to nurture with compassion. Most nurses begin their formal education with this ideal. Many nurses retain this orientation after graduation, and some manage their entire careers under this guiding principle of caring. Many of us, however, tend to forget this ideal in the hectic pace of our professional and personal lives. We may become discouraged and feel a sense of burnout.

Throughout the past decade I have spoken at many conferences with thousands of nurses. Their experience of frustration and failure is quite common. These nurses feel themselves spread as pawns across a health care system too large to control or understand. In part, this may be because they have forgotten their true roles as nurse-healers.

When individuals redirect their personal vision and empower themselves, an entire pattern may begin to change. And so it is now with the nursing profession. Most of us conceptualize nursing as much more than a vocation. We are greater than our individual roles as scientists, specialists, or care deliverers. We currently search for a name to put on our new conception of the empowered nurse. The recently introduced term *nurse-healer* aptly describes the qualities of an increasing number of clinicians, educators, administrators, and nurse practitioners. Today all nurses are awakening to the realization that they have the potential for healing.

It is my feeling that most nurses, when awakened and guided to develop their own healing potential, will function both as nurses and healers. Thus, the concept of nurse as healer is born. When nurses realize they have the ability to evoke others' healing, as well as care for them, a shift of consciousness begins to occur. As individual awareness and changes in skill building occur, a collective understanding of this new concept emerges. This knowledge, along with a shift in attitudes and new kinds of behavior, allows empowered nurses to renew themselves in an expanded role. The Nurse As Healer Series is born out of the belief that nurses are ready to embrace guidance that inspires them in their journeys of empowerment. Each book in the series may stand alone or be used in complementary fashion with other books. I hope and believe that information herein will strengthen you both personally and professionally, and provide you with the help and confidence to embark upon the path of nurse-healer.

Titles in the Nurse As Healer Series:

Healing Touch: A Resource for Health Care Professionals

Healing Life's Crises: A Guide for Nurses

The Nurse's Meditative Journal

Healing Nutrition

Healing the Dying

Awareness in Healing

Creative Imagery in Nursing

Healing and the Grief Process

Healing Addictions

D E D I C A T I O N

To my parents,
Jim and Ruth Stovall,
From whom I learned not only the joys of life
But the pain of grief

and

To my family
Bill, Shelly, and Trey
For their immeasurable love and encouragement.

Sally S. Roach

To my mom,
Amelia G. Chavez,
Whose life taught me about love
and
Whose death taught me about grief

and to my brother David, my dad Ruben, my husband
Roy, and my son Vincent
Who were there with me, through it all.

Beatriz C. Nieto

CONTENTS

P R E F A C E

Healing and the Grief Process is a practical book for all nurses in every area of nursing. Whether working in an acute care setting, an outpatient clinic, a school, or a home health agency, nurses often deal with death and dying. Those suffering the loss of a loved one are in various stages of the grieving process. Nurses with an understanding of the basic concepts of grief and a knowledge of different coping strategies are equipped with the tools necessary to guide and comfort those who need their care.

Nursing entails much more than simply working an 8-hour shift. It is a way of life. Because our professional lives are often meshed with our personal lives, we are also faced with the task of assisting those in less formal settings. Friends, co-workers, and students may turn to us for support. This book gives you basic information regarding the grieving process, identifies characteristics unique to various losses, and provides suggestions for working with clients on a formal or informal basis. Most chapters contain vignettes that provide examples from others that will furnish insight into the topic being discussed.

We believe that nurses, by virtue of their education and training, are the best possible sources for individuals to obtain the support they need as they engage in the grieving process. All nurses have the basic knowledge necessary to provide support and guidance, but they often lack confidence in their ability. With additional information on the specifics of grief and the development of certain healing characteristics in themselves, nurses can have the confidence and skills necessary to provide support and guidance to the bereaved.

As nurses, we must begin to view ourselves as healers and identify the characteristics of a nurse-healer within ourselves. As these characteristics are identified, they must be cultivated and nurtured. Enhancing and nurturing these qualities will empower us and provide us with greater joy and fulfillment in our nursing careers.

ACKNOWLEDGMENTS

Our deep appreciation and heartfelt thanks to those who shared their experiences with us and to those whom we have had the privilege of assisting in their journey though grief. Each story, each individual, each situation has provided us with insight to the uniqueness of grief and added to our personal knowledge of the grieving process.

Our heartfelt thanks to family, friends, and coworkers, especially Jayne Denham and Melva Martinez who provided editorial assistance and to MaryJo Dwyer and Malorie Garza for their research assistance.

A sincere thanks to our editor, William Burgower, to assistant editors, Debra Flis and Hilary Schrauf, and to the staff at Delmar Publishers.

A special thanks to our professor, colleague, and mentor, Lynn Keegan. Without her encouragement, this project would not have been possible.

1 | UNDERSTANDING GRIEF

Sally S. Roach and Beatriz C. Nieto

*Give sorrow words, the grief that does speak
Whispers the o'er-fraught heart and bids it break.*

Shakespeare, Macbeth (IV, iii)

When death occurs, powerful emotions are initiated that touch the deepest core of a person's being. Too often mourners are ill-prepared for such agony. Guidance is needed as they face the uncertainties of the grieving process. Nurses are frequently the health care professionals most available to provide the support and guidance needed.

Following are situations that occur in the course of a nurse's day. Each example offers a challenge and an opportunity for the nurse who has an understanding of the grieving process.

A young mother, pregnant for the second time, loses her baby six months into her pregnancy. The nurse is at the bedside as the young mother sobs.

A 25-year-old husband and father discovers that he has cancer. He is worried about the future of his family, his wife, and his three-year-old son. He turns to the nurse and cries "What am I going to do?"

A 50-year-old grandmother loses control of her car, hits the median, and runs head on into an oncoming vehicle. She arrives DOA at the Emergency Department. Her family is waiting to be told of her condition.

A staff nurse looks up from the nurses' desk and, with a heavy heart, slowly walks down the hall to answer the dying patient's call.

Nurses face loss and dying on a daily basis. If nurses are to be effective in helping others to cope with death, they must have an awareness and an understanding of their own feelings concerning grief. Knowledge of the grieving process will allow nurses to develop strategies to guide those looking to them for help through the difficult journey of grief.

DEFINITION OF TERMS

Grief

The word *grief* is derived from the Latin word *gravis*, which means heavy. The same word was later used by the French to convey that the spirits were heavy with sorrow. Grief is thought to be a normal reaction to loss. It was defined by Rando (1984) as a process of psychological, social, and somatic reactions to the perception of loss.

Grief is a universal emotion; it is inescapable and undeniable. It knows no socioeconomic boundaries and shows no cultural preference. When faced with grief, many are surprised at how powerful and painful the feelings are. Grief can be compared to being mortally wounded or severely burned. The pain is so intense and so severe that it is indescribable. As with those who have suffered burns, the healing process is long and painful and the scars remain.

Loss

Grief is an expression of intense pain resulting from a real or imagined loss. This book deals primarily with the grieving process of those who have lost a loved one. Grief, however, occurs in varying degrees with the loss of anyone or anything that an individual has a deep attachment to or values highly.

According to Rando (1984), loss is a natural part of our existence and can be categorized into two types: physical or tangible and symbolic or psychosocial. The loss of a loved one is an example of a physical loss. Examples of symbolic loss include getting a divorce or losing status because of a job demotion. The grief associated with the loss of a loved one is the main focus of this text.

Bereavement

The word *bereavement* comes from the Old English *berafian*, which means to rob, to plunder, or to dispossess. This implies that death deprives us of a continuing relationship with a loved one. In our society, the term *bereavement* refers to a separation or loss through death.

Bereavement reactions consist of the physiological, psychological, or behavioral responses to loss. Responses are individual and vary in intensity, duration, and frequency. The occurrences of these reactions comprise the bereavement process, which can persist from weeks to years.

Mourning

The word *mourn* is derived from the Old English word *murnan*, which means to express grief. Averill (1968) defined mourning as the "conventional behavior established by traditions, customs, and mores of a given society." Mourning is the expression of culturally prescribed behavior and may or may not coincide with the individual's thoughts and feelings.

GRIEF THEORIES

A number of theoretical perspectives have been proposed to identify the grieving process. None, however, has been universally accepted. Each has merit and offers insight to this complex phenomenon. Following are discussions of theories developed by Elizabeth Kübler-Ross, Erich Lindemann, John Bowlby, John Schneider, George L. Engle, and J. William Worden.

Elizabeth Kübler-Ross

Elizabeth Kübler-Ross is perhaps the most widely cited author in nursing literature concerning death and dying. In *On Death and*

Dying (1969), Kübler-Ross identified five stages of dying: denial, anger, bargaining, depression, and acceptance.

The step-by-step sequence of the Kübler-Ross model has stages that vary in length of time and often overlap. Although not absolute, the stages serve as a basis for understanding the process of dying.

The initial stage is a period of denial. The individual experiencing the loss is not ready to deal with the emotional impact of the loss. Denial is a necessary buffer; it allows time to mobilize coping abilities. Statements such as "I don't believe it," "This can't happen to me," and "You're wrong" are common in this stage.

The second emotion expressed is anger. There is a sense of outrage and resentment as denial can no longer be perpetuated. The anger is irrational and misdirected. Targets of this anger are often the nursing staff or other health care personnel, family members, or even God. Anger is an expression of the need to regain some control over the situation. Although this venting of feelings is an impetus for moving to other stages, it is important to note that anger can ebb and flow throughout the entire experience.

Bargaining is the next stage and is an attempt to postpone the inevitable. The individual seeks to negotiate a trade or make a deal: "If I can only live long enough to see my daughter graduate, then my life will be complete" or "If I can just have two more years with him, then I won't mind dying."

As the full impact of the inevitable becomes apparent, depression sets in. There is the realization that the loss is inescapable; there are no magic formulas and nothing can be done to change the situation. This stage is accompanied by overwhelming loneliness and withdrawal. The resolution of this stage leads into the final stage of acceptance.

Acceptance is a time of relative peace, not merely a grudging acceptance, but a coming to terms with the situation. At this point, individuals distance themselves from social interactions. Many patients never reach this stage of the Kübler-Ross model.

Attempts to expand the Kübler-Ross model to the grieving process have been only partially successful. Carter (1989) analyzed thirty accounts of bereavement to identify core themes related to the grieving process. In comparing the identified themes to the Kübler-Ross model, Carter concluded that essential features of bereavement identified by the participants were not addressed in the Kübler-Ross model.

Specifically, the sense of intense pain and emptiness associated with grief, as well as the desire to "hold on" to the deceased, were not addressed by Kübler-Ross. Conversely, some key features of the Kübler-Ross model had no counterpart in the grieving process. For example, no counterpart to bargaining was identified, and therefore was found to be an insignificant part of bereavement in Carter's study. The orderliness and segmentation suggested in the Kübler-Ross model was not identified as consistent with the experiences analyzed. In fact, those who had been told they would go through stages became distressed when stages could not be identified.

Elizabeth Kübler-Ross contributed greatly to the concepts of death and dying. Her writings awakened the nursing community to the needs of the dying patient. Prior to her studies, health care professionals were poorly prepared to care for the dying patient. There were few guidelines and patients were often relegated to back halls to be cared for by family members or friends. Thanks in great part to Kübler-Ross, today concepts such as death and grief are no longer ignored, but have become topics of research and literature.

Erich Lindemann

A pioneer in grief investigation, Erich Lindemann based his work on a study of the reactions of survivors and their families following the disastrous Coconut Grove Fire in Boston in 1944. In his study, Lindemann identified normal grief reactions and defined acute grief as being a normal reaction to a traumatic situation. He found that the reaction to grief could be categorized as a syndrome with psychological and somatic symptomatology. This symptomatology could appear immediately after a crisis or be delayed; it might be exaggerated or be apparently absent.

According to Lindemann (1944), the pictures portrayed by patients experiencing acute grief were remarkably similar. Because of the similarities portrayed by his patients, Lindemann was able to identify and describe what he referred to as reactions of normal grief. These reactions are discussed in the following sections.

Somatic Distress   Some examples of somatic distress that were common to Lindemann's patients included experiencing the feeling of tightness in the throat, choking, and shortness of breath. The need for sighing, a feeling of emptiness in the stomach, a lack of energy, and an intense subjective distress described as tension or mental pain were also described.

Preoccupation with the Image of the Deceased   The preoccupation occurred as a result of sensory alteration due to the traumatic loss of a loved one. The patients experienced a sense of unreality, feelings of increased emotional detachment from others, and a profound preoccupation with envisioning the deceased.

Guilt   Another strong emotion experienced by the patients was the feeling of guilt. The bereaved would dwell on the time before the death occurred and search for any shred of evidence that might indicate failure to do right by the lost loved one. Any minor oversight on the part of the bereaved was exaggerated and thought to be an act of negligence.

Hostile Reactions   Irritability, anger, and wishing to be left alone were common among the bereaved. These reactions resulted in the loss of warmth in their relationships with others.

Loss of Patterns of Conduct   Restlessness, inability to sit still, moving about in an aimless fashion, and continually searching for something to do were common complaints voiced by the bereaved.

Lindemann (1944) proposed that these five characteristics seemed to be "pathognomonic for grief" and the duration of a grief reaction depended upon the successful completion of a process known as "grief work." He described grief work as consisting of the following tasks:

- emancipation from bondage
- readjustment to the environment in which the deceased is missing
- the formation of new relationships (Lindemann, 1944, p. 143)

These stages of grief, also referred to as basic tasks of grief, have been compared to a rite of passage that the bereaved must experience and cross over in order to become completely reintegrated back into the world (Rando, 1984).

As noted earlier, Lindemann was a pioneer in the investigation of grieving. His study, however, is not without its limitations. Parks (1972) pointed out that some of these limitations include the fact that Lindemann did not provide information on the frequency of interviews, how much time had passed between the interviews, or the date the losses had occurred. Despite its limitations, Lindemann's study is an important and much-quoted piece of literature.

John Bowlby

During the 1960s, John Bowlby increased the knowledge of loss and grief through his studies on attachment. As a physician and psychoanalyst, he performed extensive clinical observations of infants and young children separated from their mothers. From these observations came the attachment theory. Bowlby concluded that attachment is a fundamental behavior that protects the survival of the individual and the species. Bowlby defined separation anxiety as a tremendous anxiety capable of producing fundamental behavior patterns that seek to restore proximity to the lost love object called the "separation response syndrome."

Bowlby (1982) differentiated separation anxiety from mourning in that separation anxiety is the response to a threat of loss of an attachment, whereas mourning is the response after a loss has occurred. Bowlby extended his attachment theory to include the grief response of bereaved adults. Grief was described as breaking the bonds of attachment. Bowlby initially identified three responses involved in the grieving process:

- yearning and searching
- disorganization and despair
- reorganization

He later added a fourth phase called numbing, which precedes yearning and searching.

The work of Bowlby was crucial in providing a better understanding of loss in children and in planning interventions with children who experience grief. His theory on adult bereavement, however, appears to be built on the work of other researchers. Because of this, it is difficult to distinguish his ideas of the grieving process in adults from those of his contemporaries.

John Schneider

The model suggested by Schneider (1984) reflected his view of grieving as being a "process of discovering the extent of what was lost and the subsequent process of discovering the extent of what was not lost or what can now take place" (p. 50). He stated that depending on the nature of the loss, the discovery process can either be all-encompassing or be brief and time limited.

Schneider introduced a theoretical model of grief that is described as holistic in nature and composed of emotional, physical, intellectual, spiritual, and behavioral aspects. This model of grief includes three themes as major tasks in the mourning process. The three themes described by Schneider include:

- limiting awareness

- awareness and perspective

- reformulation

Schneider (1984) proposed that the nature of bereavement is marked by several phases which can vary in order, intensity, and length depending on the specific loss and on each individual. The eight phases described by Schneider include:

- initial awareness

- holding on

- letting go

- awareness

- gaining perspective

- resolving loss

- reformulating loss

- transforming loss

These phases have been observed as being distinct characteristics of the tasks in the mourning process. Following are brief descriptions and examples of each of the phases.

Initial Awareness   Initial awareness usually indicates the beginning of the grief process. In describing this phase, Schneider pointed out that "it is the time when the reality of the loss reaches the conscious awareness of the individual" (p. 68). Awareness is often unanticipated, causing the person to experience both a physical and mental shock resulting from the intrusion of a new reality. This awareness can occur at the time of the loss or it can be delayed up to several years.

EXAMPLES | ***Initial Awareness***

The Nurse

After being a nurse for so many years, I still remember the first time I came face to face with a dying patient. It was an experience that I will never forget.

The Griever

It happened about a week after her funeral when I picked up the phone to call my mom that I realized she was really gone and I would never be able to talk to her again. It was like being hit with a ton of bricks.

Holding On   The holding on phase was described by Schneider as a coping strategy with "behaviors whose intent is to find some way to prevent, overcome, or reverse a loss by means of the actions or beliefs of the individual" (p. 69). Overcoming the threat or the reality of a loss is often believed to be possible by just trying hard enough.

EXAMPLES | *Holding On*

The Nurse

Let's try not to dwell so much on Mrs. Powers' death. We have other patients to care for. Let's keep busy, I always say.

The Griever

If only I had brought him to the hospital sooner; he might still be alive today.

Letting Go   The letting go phase is also seen as a coping strategy. In this phase, however, there is an attempt by the individual to downgrade the true meaning of the loss. Schneider (1984) stated that "letting go coping styles can rely on the belief that the individual is helpless in the hands of fate, God, or powerful others" (p. 69). It is during this phase that objectivity may come into play in an attempt by those in the helping professions "to maintain professional distance and to keep themselves from feeling overwhelming feelings by the sense of loss when working with dying or suffering individuals" (p. 70).

EXAMPLE | *Letting Go*

It's better to keep your distance. Don't get personally involved. You will get hurt if you do. It's not "professional" to show your feelings to a patient. You shouldn't get emotionally involved.

Awareness of Loss Awareness of loss occurs when the bereaved is no longer able to avoid the reality of the loss. He is faced with having to acknowledge that what was lost is gone and cannot be brought back, nor can it be ignored. Schneider (1984) pointed out that during this phase, the bereaved may experience feelings of helplessness, deprivation, hopelessness, and the realization of the fragility of life and that death is unavoidable. He further stated that the main purpose of this phase is to give the bereaved as much knowledge as can be tolerated regarding the significance and magnitude of the loss. It is during this phase that an individual experiences a challenge to the will to live, to physical and emotional stamina, as well as to the capacity to understand, accept, and limit feelings of helplessness.

EXAMPLES | *Awareness of Loss*

He had his whole life ahead of him. It makes you realize that it can happen to anyone at anytime.

I feel so tired, so exhausted. Will this ever end? I don't know if I can take much more of this.

Gaining Perspective There are three ways an individual may terminate the grief process. These ways are introduced in the gaining perspective phase. The first way is to return to the holding on or letting go phase. This may occur when the bereaved believes that tolerating any further pain and suffering is impossible to endure and as a result avoids dealing with the loss and is unable to complete the grief process. The second way an individual may terminate the grief process is to go through a process of healing and acceptance. The coping behaviors are replaced by resignation, acceptance, detachment, and being at peace. The bereaved lives in the present and no longer feels a sense of struggle or pain.

Schneider (1984) stated that "in terminally ill patients, this phase is often seen shortly before death and can include finishing whatever is unfinished for the individual" (p. 71).

EXAMPLE | *Gaining Perspective*

I'm ready to die. I've made peace with everyone. I have seen my children grow up and I'm thankful for my 80 years of life.

Finally, the grief process may be terminated when an individual begins to experience a motivation for change and growth. Schneider (1984) stated that at this point, the bereaved "engages in an active, usually public, step of self-forgiveness, restitution, or resolution of the loss in order to permit the reinvestment of energies elsewhere" (p. 71).

Resolving Loss   The resolving loss phase allows individuals to break away from past experiences that are now over and are no longer a part of or have a purpose in their lives. The individual may choose to go in a direction that continues to limit awareness or in a direction of acceptance. The choice of direction, as pointed out by Schneider (1984), "will depend upon how complete the awareness of the loss is, and how able the individual is to choose to resolve it" (p. 72).

EXAMPLE | *Resolving Loss*

It has taken me six years to recuperate from two almost fatal heart attacks. It was the second one that made me realize that I could die at anytime. I almost did that time. It has not been easy, but I decided to make some major changes in my life. I watch what I eat, walk two miles a day, and take more time for myself and my family. I've decided not to take my life for granted anymore.

Reformulating Loss   The reformulation phase supports the continuation of self-trust and self-awareness that results from grieving. The energy that was once spent on being bound to the past can now be used to focus on potential, growth, and new challenges. There is a feeling of freedom when the individual is able to look at a loss in a different perspective. Individuals come to terms with their own mortality and the realization that no one can count on living forever. Ralph, a nurse, cared for his father until his death. In the following vignette, Ralph relates his experience in reformulating after the loss of his father.

EXAMPLE   *Reformulating the Loss*

When I took care of my dying father, I couldn't understand why he had to suffer so and why I had to be the one caring for him. Well, now that I think about it, his death taught me so much about what really matters in life. Things like family, love, trust, companionship, and that death is just a part of life that everyone must experience. From this experience, I feel I can better help others deal with a death and loss of a loved one.

Transforming Loss   The main purpose of this last phase, according to Schneider (1984), is to "permit individuals to be open to all experiences and sources of knowledge and to be in a perspective of life that is not bound by physical mortality, societal imperatives, or their sensory apparatus, but which includes and expands on these" (p. 74). It is during this phase that the person views the loss as part of life and that the grief is a unifying rather than an alienating human experience. The following example illustrates how one nurse transformed the loss of a patient and gained a greater insight into death.

EXAMPLE   *Transforming Loss*

It took me awhile to realize that I am not the only one that has ever suffered the loss of a patient. Going through this loss has been a growing experience and I no longer need to see myself as special for experiencing it. I can now accept that I experienced an event that others have gone through in the past and others will experience in the future.

George L. Engle

According to Engle (1964), grief is the "typical reaction to the loss of a source of psychological gratification" (p. 94). Sources of psychological gratification include such "love objects" as a parent, a spouse, a child, a friend, a job, a pet, and so on.

Engle identified three stages involved in the mourning process:

- shock and disbelief
- developing awareness
- restitution and resolution

Progress through these stages is necessary if healing is to occur. Although there is progression from one stage to another, there is also movement within each stage.

The initial stage is shock and disbelief. Reactions vary and range from crying out, fainting, and pacing to the inability to speak. The individual feels disoriented and helpless. This may be followed by a numbing or lack of feeling where the person may sit motionless and dazed. During this stage, a "searching for the lost love" can occur. "I thought I saw her" or "I keep expecting her to wake me up and tell me it's a dream" or "I see him everywhere; then he turns around and it's not him." Denial is a part of this stage of mourning and can serve as a useful avenue to buffer the shock until the individual is able to face the reality of the situation. This stage may last from a few minutes to several days.

Often within hours, Engle's second stage of developing awareness begins. The reality of the loss penetrates the consciousness, causing great psychological pain. Overwhelming feelings of loss and helplessness occur. The realization that the individual is powerless to change the circumstances of the loss contributes to the pain.

Anger and hostility may surface and may be expressed toward family members or health care professionals. Feelings of guilt may also surface. Guilt from the manner in which the griever behaved or the perception that she in some way contributed to the death may cause a great deal of pain. Sadness, isolation, and loneliness may also be present.

Some shed tears, others are unable to and must either wait until they are alone or cry inwardly. Tears are socially acceptable for those who grieve and crying appears to be a form of communication that elicits support and help from those seeking to comfort the griever. According to Engle, this stage may last from six months to one year.

The last stage, restitution and recovery, is the longest stage, and can last up to several years. This stage marks the beginning of the healing process. According to Engle, restitution is the true work of mourning. Rituals and customs such as the funeral, family gatherings, and viewing the body initiate the recovery process. These activities force denial to the surface. The reality of death can no longer be denied. As the reality of death becomes accepted, the process of resolution proceeds.

According to Engle, bodily pains appear in place of the numbness experienced in the first stage. Thoughts are predominantly on the deceased. The deceased may be idealized and all negative attitudes repressed. With time, the identification with the ideals and aspirations of the lost love provides the incentive to resume living. The goal of this stage is to accept the loss and surrender the lost love. New relationships and new patterns of social interaction must develop. The lost love is not forgotten, but the griever begins to come to terms with the loss. The pain is less severe, ambivalent feelings are tolerated, and new relationships and social patterns are initiated.

The grieving process is not a gradual, one-way process, but rather a series of ups and downs, exacerbations, and regressions. For the mourner, this process can be difficult since outwardly life seems normal, but inwardly the mourner is coming to grips with the loss. While society is lenient and even encourages outward expressions of grief early in the grieving process, in the later stages, outward expressions of grief are not tolerated as well.

Successful resolution has occurred when the mourner has the ability to remember both positive and negative aspects of the lost relationship and make and sustain new relationships. Engle emphasized that mourning may continue for several years and the process cannot be accelerated. Lai-Chu's experience with grief illustrates Engle's theory.

Lai-Chu's Experience with Grief

Shock and Disbelief

Lai-Chu, a young girl of 14, was sitting motionless in the Emergency Department waiting room. Her heart felt like it was going to explode. She wanted to cry, but the tears wouldn't come. All she could think about was the picture of her mother lying helpless on the floor when she came in from school. The sounds of the ambulance, the questioning, the ride to the hospital all rolled over and over in her head. How could this happen to her? She needed her mother so much. Her dad came and he was frightened too, but Lai-Chu felt so numb. Then the doctor came and said, "I'm sorry. We did all we could, but it was no use, her heart did not respond." Lai-Chu immediately began crying with uncontrollable sobs. She felt like the floor had fallen out from under her. How could she make it without her mom? What would she do?

Developing Awareness

Over the next several days, the pain Lai-Chu felt was overwhelming, the sadness unbearable, and a feeling of total helplessness prevailed. She was angry at the doctors for not saving her mother, yet at the same time she felt that, maybe, if she had done something different, her mother would still be alive. "Mom worried so much about me. At times we argued over what time I should come home, my choice of friends, or school work. If only I had not been so selfish, wanting my own way..."

Restitution and Recovery

Everyone was there. The church was so crowded. Lai-Chu and the rest of the family sat, crying quietly. Surprisingly, the friends who were present, those who took time to come to the funeral, provided so much comfort. To know that so many people cared about her mother and her family felt good. Strange how it comforted her. As the months came and went, Lai-Chu slowly began to feel again. In fact, the numbness she felt in the beginning gave way to headaches that were only relieved by sleep. Emotions ebbed and flowed. Thoughts of her mother permeated her being all the time and she talked about her "great mother" in glowing terms. After 10 months of emotional ups and downs, Lai-Chu slowly began to resume living again. Her grades improved, and she began to enjoy social activities and "hanging around" with her friends again. One day, when she was alone and thinking about her mother, she suddenly knew what her mother would want. She would want her to be truly alive and happy. Aloud she said, "I love you, Mom, forever and ever! But I must go on. I can be happy again."

Lai-Chu's expressions indicated that, while her love had not diminished, she was beginning to recover from the painful experience of losing her mother.

J. William Worden

As assistant professor of psychology at Harvard Medical School and research director of Massachusetts General Hospital's Omega Project, William Worden (1982) has been involved in a series of longitudinal studies on life-threatening illness and life-threatening behavior. Basing his work on the work done by Lindemann in 1944, Worden was able to observe similarities in the behavior exhibited by his patients experiencing an acute grief reaction and those studied by Lindemann 40 years prior to his own work.

Worden's studies (as cited in Cooley, 1992) identified four major tasks that an individual must accomplish before successful adjustment to the loss occurs. Worden believed that the individual must:

- accept the reality of the loss

- experience the pain of grief

- adjust to an environment in which the deceased is missing

- withdraw emotional energy and reinvest it in another relationship

There are a number of behaviors that might be exhibited by an individual experiencing an acute grief reaction. Because the list of behaviors is so extensive and varied, Worden grouped these behaviors into four general categories:

- feelings

- physical sensations

- cognition or thought processes

- behaviors

These behaviors are referred to as manifestations of normal grief (see table 1.1). Not all of these behaviors, however, will be experienced by one person.

Worden (1982) pointed out that "it is important for bereavement counselors to understand the wide range of behaviors covered under normal grief so they will not pathologize behavior that should be recognized as normal" (p. 28). Having an adequate understanding of these behaviors and experiences will also

Feelings		Physical Sensations
Sadness	Anger	Hollowness in stomach
Guilt	Yearning	Sensitivity to noise
Relief	Numbness	Tightness in the chest or throat
Emancipation	Helplessness	Depersonalization
Self-reproachment	Shock	Shortness of breath
Anxiety	Loneliness	Muscular weakness
Fatigue		Lethargy
		Dry mouth

Behaviors	Cognition or Thought Process
Crying	Disbelief
Sleep disorders	Sense of presence
Absentmindedness	Confusion
Dreams of the deceased	Hallucinations
Restlessness	Preoccupation
Appetite disturbances	
Social withdrawal	
Avoiding reminders of the deceased	
Treasuring objects belonging to the deceased	

TABLE 1.1 *Manifestations of Normal Grief*

From *Grief Counseling and Grief Therapy: A Handbook for the Mental Health Practitioner*, by J. William Worden, 1982, New York: Springer Publishing Co., Inc. Copyright 1982 by Springer Publishing Co., Inc. Reprinted by permission.

"enable counselors to give reassurance to people experiencing such behaviors as disturbing, especially in the case of a first significant loss" (p. 28).

ATTRIBUTES OF GRIEF

A review of current and classic literature regarding grief was done by Cowles and Rodgers (1991). Their intent was to expand and clarify the definition of grief. Their findings revealed five attributes of grief: process, individualized, dynamic, pervasive, and normative. These findings assist in the conceptualization of grief.

Grief Is a Process

Grief is presented as having phases of activity described by Lindemann (1944) as "grief work." This work takes time, often a considerable amount of time, and sometimes the griever never reaches a point where the grief work is totally complete. The idea of a process rather than stages is more appropriate since stages imply a neat progression with an identifiable beginning and ending. Grief, however, is somewhat messy, with the griever experiencing and re-experiencing emotions thought to be under control. The process, while somewhat predictable, is also highly individual. To adhere to a rigid time frame or stages can be counter-productive since the success of grief work can most appropriately be determined by the griever's acceptance of the loss and ability to go on with life.

Grief Is Individualized

The grief experience is highly individual and is influenced by a number of variables: the nature of the loss, the relationship between those involved, previous coping mechanisms, the effectiveness of a support system, and religious and cultural background. The individual's life experiences and previous experience with loss also play an important role. These variables affect each individual differently and each individual reacts accordingly.

Grief Is Dynamic

While grief appears to have identifiable phases, the individual moves continuously through phases during the grief experience. The griever may feel successful in certain areas only to feel suddenly overcome with emotions thought to be under control. Many are surprised by the vigorous and powerful emotions that confront the mourner. Grief requires tremendous amounts of energy and can leave those who mourn totally drained.

Grief Is Pervasive

Grief permeates every aspect of the mourner's life: physical, spiritual, and emotional. It is holistic in nature. The very essence of the individual's being is tested.

Grief Is Normative

All individuals face common emotions; for example, love, anger, and fear. Each emotion gives meaning to our lives and provides an avenue for growth. Grief is one of these normal emotions. Terms used when grief follows a predictable or expected path are *normal* or *uncomplicated* grief. Although it is most often a normal process, grief that continues too long or extends beyond social or cultural expectations becomes *pathological* or *complicated* grief.

CONSENSUS ON THE DEFINITION OF GRIEF

All of the early studies on the grieving process and most of the current studies have been done by medical doctors, psychologists, and sociologists. Even with the past and present research, there is no consensus on the definition of grief or the grieving process. The concept of grief continues to be ambiguous and vague. Nursing knowledge concerning grief has been gleaned from other disciplines. Only within the last 20 years has any significant nursing research that focuses on grief and bereavement been done. The majority of nursing research seeks to add to the knowledge and conceptualization of grief in order to clarify this important phenomenon.

The authors take an eclectic approach to dealing with grief. Just as there are no neat, well-formed linear stages to grief, no single theory provides the complete framework for the individualistic and dynamic process of grief. The eclectic approach allows the mourner to progress through grief without the pressure of being forced to grieve in a preconceived format or in the "correct" manner.

THE ROLE OF THE NURSE IN THE GRIEVING PROCESS

Nurses are in a unique position to intervene in the initial phases of grief and to offer support and guidance as the process continues. The nurse's role is one of support, guidance, and teacher. Since individuals respond to grief based on their background and coping styles, nurses must be sensitive and intuitive in assessing and recognizing the symptomatology involved in the grieving process.

The loss the client experiences is a wound that must heal. The grieving process is the method of healing. Contemporary nurses are expanding their knowledge to recognize that they are healers. When grief is viewed as a wound that must heal, the nurse becomes the guide in facilitating the healing process.

Dossey et al. (1988) described the role of the nurse-healer as one who "helps others discover and recognize new health behaviors, make choices and discover insights about how to cope effectively" (p. 42). Guiding is a special art and intervention that nurses can use to assist the client to be in harmony with inner resources, decrease stress, and explore meaning and purpose in life (Dossey et al., 1988). Future chapters will include specific aspects of the role of the nurse-healer in guiding the client through the bereavement process.

SUMMARY

Nurses are confronted with loss and dying on a daily basis. They are often the first health care professionals to have the opportunity to intervene in times of crisis. A knowledge of the grieving process will enable the nurse to intercede appropriately. Appropriate intercession provides the support and care needed by those who suffer the emotional pain of the death of a loved one. This chapter presents an overview of the most prominent theories of grief by the following theorists: Elizabeth Kübler-Ross, Erich Lindemann, John Bowlby, John Schneider, George Engle, and William Worden.

While much has been written about grief, there is no consensus on the definition of grief. The concept continues to be ambiguous and vague. Regardless of the stages or phases of grief, the process can be painful. Intervention by the nurse often helps to ease the pain. Nurses who perceive themselves as an adjunct to the healing process become nurse-healers. Nurse-healers are able to provide guidance and insight to the griever and facilitate the healing process.

REFLECTIONS

1. Think about the losses you have suffered. How have they affected your nursing practice?

2. In what ways are you able to facilitate healing in the grieving patient?

3. Do you shy away from those who are grieving?

4. How do your experiences with grief relate to the theories postulated in this chapter?

References

Averill, J. R. (1968). Grief: Its nature and significance. *Psychological Bulletin, 70,* 721–748.

Bowlby, J. (1982). *Attachment and loss: Vol. 2, Separation anxiety and anger.* New York: Basic Books, Inc.

Carter, S. (1989, November/December). Themes of grief. *Nursing Research, 38*(6), 354–358.

Cooley, M. E. (1992). Bereavement care: A role for nurses. *Cancer Nursing, 15*(2), 125–129.

Cowles, K. V., & Rodgers, B. L. (1991). The concept of grief: A foundation for nursing research and practice. *Research in Nursing and Health, 14*, 119–127.

Dossey, B., Keegan, L., Guzzetta, C., & Kolkmeier, L. (1988). *Holistic nursing: A handbook for practice.* Gaithersburg, MD: Aspen Publishers, Inc.

Engle, G. (1964, September). Grief and grieving. *American Journal of Nursing, 64*(9), 93–98.

Kübler-Ross, E. (1969). *On death and dying.* New York: The Macmillan Co.

Lindemann, E. (1944). Symptomatology and management of acute grief. *American Journal of Psychiatry, 101*, 141–148.

Parks, C. M. (1972). *Bereavement: Studies of grief in adult life.* New York: International Universities Press.

Rando, T. A. (1984). *Grief, dying and death: Clinical interventions for caregivers.* Champaign, IL: Research Press Company.

Schneider, J. (1984). *Stress, loss and grief: Understanding their origins and growth potential.* Baltimore: University Park Press.

Worden, J. W. (1982). *Grief counseling and grief therapy: A handbook for the mental health professional.* New York: Springer Publishing Co.

2 ANTICIPATORY GRIEF

Beatriz C. Nieto

> *But the waiting time, my brothers,*
> *Is the hardest time of all.*

Sarah Doudney

In the first chapter, some major theorists and their concepts on grieving, loss, and bereavement were introduced. The type of loss that someone experiences will determine the type of grieving that will take place. There are basically three major categories of grief. First, there is the grief that occurs before a death, as in terminal illness. Second, there is the grief that occurs after the death from a chronic illness. Third, there is the grief that occurs after a sudden and unexpected death, as in accidents, murders, suicides, or heart attacks.

In this chapter, anticipatory grief and the effects it has on the dying patient, the family, and the nurse are discussed. Along with factual information regarding anticipatory grief, actual accounts written by individuals who have experienced the anticipation of someone's death and strategies that facilitate coping are presented.

DEFINITION OF ANTICIPATORY GRIEF

The term *anticipatory grief* was first coined by Erich Lindemann in 1944 when he used the phrase to refer to "the emotional reaction that occurs before an expected loss" (Stephenson, 1985, p. 158). Although the concept of anticipatory grief was introduced over 50 years ago, its significance today continues to be very important because people are living longer, have longer terminal illnesses, and are dying more frequently of chronic diseases.

The use of state-of-the-art medical technology has brought us to the age of predicting when death can and will take place. This forewarning of death to families is more common now than ever before and is a major contributor to the state of anticipation known as anticipatory grief. Anticipatory grief can be experienced by all involved, including the dying patient. Rando (1984) stated that anticipatory grief "is a form of normal grief that occurs in the anticipation of a future loss" and that it is "the term most often used when discussing the families of the terminally ill" (p. 37).

SYMPTOMS AND PROCESSES

The symptoms and processes of grief following a loss are also a part of anticipatory grief. Fulton and Fulton (1971) identified the following to be integral factors that come into play when an individual is experiencing anticipatory grief: (1) depression, (2) heightened concern for the terminally ill person, (3) rehearsal of the death, and (4) attempts to adjust to the consequences of the death. They went on to say that the main functions of anticipatory grief are to allow the family to: (1) absorb the reality of the loss gradually over time, (2) finish unfinished business with the dying person, (3) begin to change assumptions about life and identity, and (4) make plans for the future so that they will not feel betrayed by the deceased after death.

Conceptualizing Anticipatory Grief

A study by Futterman, Hoffmann, and Sabshin (1972) concluded that acknowledgment, grieving, reconciliation, detachment, and memorialization were major aspects of conceptualizing anticipatory grief. Although their study was based on parental anticipatory grief, these conceptualizing aspects may be applicable to anticipatory grief in general. These aspects are described as follows:

Acknowledgment During this time, the parents are becoming progressively convinced that the child's death is inevitable.

Grieving The parents are experiencing and expressing the emotional impact of the anticipated loss and the physical, psychological, and interpersonal turmoil associated with it.

Reconciliation During the reconciliation period, the parents are developing perspectives on the child's expected death. This preserves a sense of confidence in the worth of the child's life and in the worth of life in general.

Detachment There is the withdrawing of emotional investment from the child as a growing being with a real future.

Memorialization The parents develop a fixed conscious mental representation of the dying child that will endure beyond her death (p. 252).

These conceptual aspects of anticipatory grief are applicable to anyone experiencing the anticipation of a loved one's death, whether young or old.

PHASES OF ANTICIPATORY GRIEF

Anticipatory grief is similar to the typical grief process in the sense that how a person grieves is determined by several factors, including, but not limited to:

- the personality of the individual experiencing the loss; his emotional and physical well-being
- the nature of the relationship
- the social context in which the loss is taking place

The initial phase of the typical grief process and that of anticipatory grief involves the reaction to the news of the impending loss. When a loved one is diagnosed as terminal, the initial reactions experienced by the individuals may include shock and disbelief. It is during this time that they are full of questions like *Why did it have to happen? How could this happen to her, to us? What is going to happen now? How long does she have to live? What do we do now? Is there any hope?* Hope? Yes, hope. The uniqueness of anticipatory grief is that although the initial reaction by those involved is shock and disbelief, the feeling of hope plays an important part in anticipatory grief as well. Because the loss has not yet occurred, the individuals faced with an impending death may still hope that all will be well. Hope involves the feeling that somehow their loved one will not die, but be cured and have the opportunity to live a long, happy, and productive life.

There is a vast fluctuation of emotions that may be displayed by individuals experiencing anticipatory grief. These fluctuations of emotions can be described as an emotional roller coaster ride because like a roller coaster ride, an individual's emotional status is subjected to many ups and downs. First there are the ups, when the dying person is feeling well enough to participate in everyday activities with the other members of his family. During this time, he can eat, talk, and stay up a little longer without getting tired. Making plans for the future is not clouded over by feelings of pain, anger, or frustration. The ups are the times when there are periods of remissions, good days, and progress toward obtaining health seems possible.

Then come the downs, when it seems the pain will never subside. Feelings of hopelessness and uselessness emerge because there is nothing more the individual can do to relieve the loved one's pain. Anger and impatience at the person for being ill and at herself for feeling so helpless may appear. It is at this point that individuals are faced with the reality of increasing physical degeneration, worsening symptoms, and having to make decisions to use more "heroic" medical measures to help the dying person.

Needless to say, this emotional roller coaster ride can and does take a toll on all who are involved with the impending death. The hardest part of all, however, is not knowing when the ride will end.

The second phase of grief has been identified as the period of disorganization and reorganization. According to Stephenson

(1985) this is the phase in which the individual will most typically remain during anticipatory grief. It is during this phase that the individual faced with impending death comes to the realization that death is a reality. Time once thought to be limitless now becomes limited. There is an indescribable heaviness to the finiteness that seems to linger over all those who wait. Becker (1973) claimed that although attempts are made to deceive ourselves by thinking that things will last forever, that death will not touch us, the diagnosis of terminality brings us face-to-face with the reality of death; a reality that we have fought so hard to deny.

The ambiguity of feelings that is so apparent in the initial phase continues throughout the second phase of anticipatory grief as well. The individual experiencing anticipatory grief is caught between trying to meet his own needs and helping to meet the needs of the dying person. It is during this time that the individual feels the pressure of having to care for a dying loved one and keep up with his own obligations as well. The family member may feel that time spent away from the dying person is time lost. Time is no longer limitless. Individuals facing the loss of a loved one are often confronted with wanting to spend as much time with the dying person while simultaneously striving to keep some normalcy in their own lives. The caregiver may ponder questions such as *Shouldn't I spend as much time as possible with her? What if something happens and I'm not there?* At the same time, concern over how much time can be taken away from other obligations and other roles begins to emerge. Much to our dismay, questions to which there are no cut and dry answers must be faced.

BENEFITS OF ANTICIPATORY GRIEF

Even though it is never an easy journey for the person experiencing anticipatory grief, the journey does have some beneficial aspects that are noteworthy. Some of the major benefits that anticipatory grief allows for are: giving both the bereaved to be and the dying person the opportunity to tie up loose ends, to resolve interpersonal issues that need to be taken care of, to make amends, and to prepare. It may also provide the time to resolve the questions of existential grief and allow time to prepare to deal with the impending death. Of course, to what extent anyone can prepare himself for someone's death is difficult to determine.

From interviews of parents whose children had died of cancer, Rando (1984) concluded that the optimal length for anticipatory grief is from 6 to 18 months. She found that a shorter amount of time did not give the parents the opportunity to prepare for the loss. A longer period of time, however, often had a debilitating effect. She further concluded that the longer the illness, the greater the anger and the number of atypical responses found among the sample in her study.

Successful Anticipatory Grief

According to Stephenson (1985), "successful anticipatory grief means being aware of the disorganization that is occurring and learning to live with it" (p. 160). He also said that "to be involved in anticipatory grief means to acknowledge and live with death; to acknowledge one's inability to master it, and one's ultimate helpless position in the world" (p. 161). Though no one wishes to think of death, many must come to grips with the reality of the impending death of a loved one. Truly, the anticipation of someone's death is never easy. This is true for the family and also the person who is dying. The family is coming face to face with losing one of its members. On the other hand, the dying person is faced with losing every earthly relationship. There will be a multitude of distinct emotions and feelings experienced by both the dying person and her family. The degree to which these emotions and feelings vary will depend on the amount of time they have together before the death occurs. It is no wonder that many feel so ill-equipped to deal with such a traumatic situation.

Responses to Anticipatory Grief

The following stories are true accounts taken from a journal kept by a nurse whose mother was diagnosed with metastatic breast cancer over a year ago. The first excerpt was written by the nurse approximately six months after her mother was diagnosed with breast cancer. In this excerpt, some of the feelings and emotions that occur in anticipatory grief are brought to light. The second excerpt was written by the mother just a few months before her death occurred. The third excerpt was written by the hospice nurse who was involved with their care. They were willing to share some excerpts from their journals to help others realize the devastation felt when someone you love is diagnosed as terminal.

The Daughter

Even when I am not there with her physically, I'm there with her spiritually, mentally. I find myself thinking of her, suddenly wondering if she is doing as well as when I last saw her, which was only a few hours ago. Who would have ever thought that I would be having to use all my skills as a nurse to make sure that her pain and suffering will be minimized and that her death will be peaceful. How awful this all sounds. I can't remember the day when I didn't think my mom would never grow old, would never get sick, and somehow would always remain the strong, vibrant, active person she had always been. To see her now, wasted down to practically nothing, is so devastating. Yet, that little spark in her eyes, that lets me know that her spirit is still alive, remains. Maybe, just maybe, she will pull through. The hospice nurses are amazed at how well she has been responding to her treatments. Maybe there is still hope that she will survive. For now we live for the good moments and I say moments because the days seem to get longer and longer and the waiting gets worse and worse. How we depended on her, how she was there for all of us. She was always there, for whoever needed help. Even now we want her to be there, but she is so tired, so very tired. But why does she hang on? How much more can her body, soul, and spirit take? She has gone through so much; we have all gone through so much. Yet, we are all grateful for each day she is with us. I really don't know what I would do or will do without her. I'll never forget her, that is for sure. I'll never forget how our relationship got stronger, even though it was because of her illness. For this I am thankful. Now she needs me to take care of her and this has made our relationship more intimate. But why did it have to happen to her, WHY MY MOM?? I guess I will never know the answer to that question, but I do know that I thank God I am able to help her. For now, we have to live day by day and enjoy her while she is still with us.

The Patient

I ask the Lord why he keeps me here like this. I feel I am nothing but trouble to my family. I know they are getting tired of having to take care of me. I try but I can no longer do anything for myself. Heaven knows I try, but my strength has left me. I am ready to go, but I know that I have to wait until the Lord calls me. I've made peace with my family and have told them to put me into God's hand. It is so hard to watch them look at me. I know I don't look like I did just a few months ago. I look in the mirror at myself and can hardly believe that is me looking back. I feel so old and tired. Everything is failing me. How can this be happening to me? What will become of my family? Oh Lord, in heaven, I pray that you take care of my family and that you take me soon.

The Nurse

I have been a hospice nurse for several years now, and dealing with someone's death is never easy. Every patient is special and so courageous. It is hard to forget those that I have taken care of. Those that have shared with me an event, so intimate, and so taboo to many. I know that dealing with death and dying is part of my job, but sometimes it does take its toll on me.

COPING

Words cannot express the devastation felt when a family member or loved one is diagnosed as terminal. The news goes through your body like a shock wave, numbing you until it seems that you are living in a daze and in a cloud of fog that never seems to lift. You try everything within your power; finding the best doctors, hospitals, latest medical treatments, and so on, for your loved one. You keep up with all their appointments. You go to one hospital for tests and to the other hospital for radiation treatments. The doctors, in the meantime, say, "She's holding her own, her blood work looks better," yet she keeps losing weight.

You keep this up until one day you find yourself driving around with your loved one, not knowing where to go or what to do next. It seems that though you keep up with the treatments prescribed, something else seems to go wrong. Now she is having more trouble breathing. She is no longer continent of urine since her radiation treatments. It seems she is growing weaker and weaker by the minute. You keep thinking that she can't die like this. You know that if you take her to the hospital they will want to admit her, hook her up to all sorts of machines, and run all sorts of tests again. You know you do not want her to be put through that because those machines and tests will not cure her or make her better. You know this, but you do not know what else to do, so you wind up in the emergency room anyway. As you predicted, they hook her up to all sorts of monitors and routine blood work is ordered as well. You ask the doctor if it is necessary that an EKG or an IV or lab work be done. She is terminal you know. He tells you that this is their job and if you did not want this done, you should not have brought her to the emergency room.

But where do I take her? She is so weak, what do I do now? Just when you think that there is no help available and that you are totally alone, a nurse says, "What you need is hospice." Hospice? I've heard of that, but I do not know anything about it. Then the nurse tells you that she recently lost her father after a long-term illness. She tells you that after going through what you are experiencing at this point, she was introduced to hospice by a fellow nurse. It had made a tremendous difference in the care of her father. You listen, and as you listen you begin to realize that you and your loved one can have some control about what is to happen and that control can be facilitated.

Guiding and Supporting the Family's Decision

This account is an example of how we as nurses, no matter where our place of employment happens to be, are in a unique position to help both the family and the dying patient in their hour of need. The emergency room nurse used her skills and past experience to assess the situation. She took the opportunity to bring a new perspective to the situation by giving the family an alternate way to care for the dying patient. In this situation, the family decided to use hospice as the method of care for their terminally ill loved one. Others may not feel comfortable with this type of care. These families may want the use of technological heroics for their loved one. They may choose to do everything possible to prolong their loved one's life. In either case, we need to be sensitive to the needs of each individual situation. This will enable us to be instrumental in guiding and supporting whatever decision the family and/or patient may make.

In order for nurses to guide and support these families, we need to feel comfortable with our own feelings about death and dying. We need to monitor our own feelings and know that we are not immune to sadness, anxiety, or the need to express personal concern. We have to realize that our reactions to given situations are conditioned by our own experiences with earlier losses. This may include our ability to handle angry or hostile reactions of others, whether they are a friend, patient, student, or family member. We need to educate ourselves to be well-informed about what support groups and programs are available for the dying patient and the family.

As nurses we need to be ourselves and say what we feel. Death is a subject that is never easy to talk about and "has a way of sealing people off, making them feel totally isolated" (Bertman, 1991, p. 198). We need to realize that we are human, with human emotions. In sharing our feelings, we can reestablish our connection with others.

To help bring this into perspective, Callanan (1994) outlined some steps that might aid in alleviating the discomfort of nurses when faced with death and dying. They are as follows:

Consider Your Own Feelings We, as nurses, need to search within ourselves and find our true feelings and/or fears concerning death and dying, and then acknowledge that they exist. We need to keep in mind that our fears may be different from those of our patients. Our focus should be on their needs rather than our own.

Understand the Patient and How He Copes We need to look at the person as an individual having his own way of dealing with stress and loss. Consider whether the person is a quiet, introspective man or an inquisitive extrovert. This is important to know because the patient's usual behavior may intensify in the face of his terminal illness. If he is normally quiet, the patient may become more so and may seem withdrawn. On the other hand, if the patient is normally an extrovert, he may be seen as more demanding. What we need to keep in mind is that these reactions are normal and healthy for him; therefore, they should be respected, and not challenged.

Open the Door to Communication The key element for facilitating communication with the patient is timing. A few minutes in the morning might not be the best time for the patient, but it might give you the opportunity to mutually agree on a time that would allow for a more meaningful discussion.

Consider What the Patient Knows It is possible that a patient may not know or understand the seriousness of her condition. The best way to find out is to ask her to tell you about her illness. Use general terms such as "illness" instead of specific disease names like "cancer" when talking to the patient. You may also want to use the words the patient uses to describe her condition until you can pinpoint exactly what she knows.

Answering Difficult Questions   Patients may want to know what it feels like to die. They may fear having to endure much pain and suffering throughout the course of their illness. We need to be honest and direct when answering their questions. We need to stress to them that all the necessary steps will be taken to assure their comfort level will be maintained.

Honest Concern and Support   We have to realize that our patients do not expect us to have all the answers to their questions. There are so many questions about death and dying that are not answerable. What they do want, need, and expect from us is our honest concern, support, and above all, our willingness to listen and to help if we can.

FACILITATING GRIEVING

Rando (1984) pointed out that "what the griever needs most are acceptance and nonjudgmental listening which will facilitate the expression of emotions and the necessary review of the relationship with the lost loved one" (p. 79). To help the griever, the nurse can intervene in many ways. One of the most important interventions that nurses can use is the giving of themselves. Their presence and concern for the family can aid in facilitating the grieving process. Knowing that there is another source of support, the family may feel that they are not alone and that they are not expected to handle the situation on their own. There is nothing worse than thinking that you and you alone are responsible for the dying person.

Encouraging the verbalization of feelings by the family and the dying patient is another important way to facilitate grieving. This may be done by providing reassurance that they are not going crazy or having a breakdown, and that the acute pain they are feeling is part of the grieving process. Encourage them to talk about what is happening; to cry, or even scream if necessary, and assure them that these feelings are normal and expected in this type of situation.

The important thing to remember is to abstain from being judgmental or critical of how others handle their grief. There is no painless way to go through the grief process. As nurses, we can help the family realize that "although the pain may be distressing, the experience and release of it is a healing part of that process" (Rando, 1984, p. 98).

SUMMARY

Bertman (1991) stated that grief is love not wanting to let go and that it can be likened to a "blow" or a cut in which the wound gradually heals. She also said that grief may make us vulnerable, both physically and emotionally, and that it might even disable us temporarily. Working through it, however, will ultimately make us stronger. We, as nurses, need to keep in mind that grief is not a disease. Grief is a normal process that allows individuals to cope with a loss, no matter what that loss may be. We need to remember that grief is a unique and individualized experience, varying from one person to another and that we need to be supportive and nonjudgmental when dealing with the grieving individual.

REFLECTIONS

1. Think about some of the most difficult situations that you have had to deal with in your life.

2. Have any of these situations involved a loss? If so, was it a physical or a symbolic loss? Or did your loss involve the death of a significant other or loved one?

3. How did you react at the time you were faced with the situation?

4. Think about your reactions after you dealt with the situation and since then.

5. Can you relate to some of the situations presented in this chapter? Have you become more aware of the needs of the grieving individual?

References

Becker, E. (1973). *The denial of death.* New York: The Free Press.

Bertman, S. L. (1991). *Facing death: Images, insights, and interventions. A handbook for educators, healthcare professionals, and counselors.* New York: Hemisphere Publishing Corporation.

Callanan, M. (1994). Breaking the silence: What to do when you feel your terminally ill patient wants to talk about death, but you're not sure how to open a dialogue. *American Journal of Nursing, 94*(1), 22–23.

Fulton, R., & Fulton, J. (1971). A psychosocial aspect of terminal care: Anticipatory grief. *Omega, 2,* 91–92.

Futterman, E. H., Hoffman, I., & Sabshin, M. (1972). Parental anticipatory mourning. In B. Schoenberg, A. C. Carr, D. Peretz, & A. H. Kutscher (Eds.), *Psychological management in medical practice.* New York: Columbia University Press.

Rando, T. A. (1984). *Grief, dying, and death: Clinical interventions for caregivers.* Champaign, IL: Research Press Company.

Stephenson, J. S. (1985). *Death, grief, and mourning: Individual and social realities.* New York: The Free Press.

3 THE ROLE OF HOSPICE

Sally S. Roach

*Those who have the strength and the love to sit
with a dying patient in the silence that goes
beyond words will know that this moment is neither
frightening nor painful, but a peaceful cessation
of the functioning of the body.*

Elizabeth Kübler-Ross

Death and dying are often accompanied by a conspiracy of silence and avoidance. Physicians, nurses, family, and friends, as well as the terminally ill patient, contribute to this conspiracy. The fear of saying the wrong thing, uncertainty of what the patient knows about her condition, and each person's fear of his own mortality all influence this conspiracy. Silence and avoidance are self-protective measures of escaping the reality of terminal illness. These measures allow no interaction, no growth, and no peace, only fear and uncertainty.

Nurses and physicians have long upheld the medical model of health care. Healing measures are disregarded and curative measures are emphasized. In the minds of many medically minded health professionals, if a cure is unattainable, then failure is the only alternative. Health care professionals perpetuate the medical model myth by avoiding the patient and the family and maintaining the silence. Unfortunately, this avoidance does nothing to alleviate the pain and suffering of the patient or the family. The following vignette illustrates the lack of support given by the nursing staff to Jo Beth as she faced death.

Jo Beth's Battle

Jo Beth had been fighting cancer for over five years. The first symptom was a lump in her breast that proved to be malignant. She had a mastectomy, followed by radiation therapy and chemotherapy. Four years later, the cancer that had begun in her breast had metastasized to her lungs and brain. She was growing weaker by the day. Her husband had left her three years before. Her two daughters, ages 14 and 19, were almost as frightened as she was. She turned to her friend, Sue. Together they discussed the cancer that had so relentlessly taken control of her life. They discussed her fear of death. Sue assured Jo Beth that she would be available whenever she needed her.

Jo Beth could almost feel her body growing weaker each day. Breathing was difficult and the pain was severe. One day Jo Beth called Sue crying hysterically. She was desperately afraid and unable to breathe. Was she going to die in front of her children?

Sue, Jo Beth, and her two daughters rushed frantically to the hospital. At the Emergency Department they waited several hours, but the physician was reluctant to admit Jo Beth to the hospital saying there was nothing he could do for her. Jo Beth was desperately afraid of dying. The nurse was arranging for her dismissal when Sue intervened. "Nurse, you can see that Jo Beth is suffering and she is so weak she cannot walk. She needs to be here where she can be made comfortable if nothing else. Isn't there something you can do?" The nurse shook her head and left. After a short while, she returned with a slight smile on her face. The Emergency Department doctor had agreed to admit Jo Beth to the hospital for 24 hours of "observation." In the hospital, Jo Beth and her daughters had minimal contact with the staff. The nurses were polite but formal and distant. Jo Beth died 23 hours later in a hospital room with her two daughters and Sue at her side.

This situation should never have occurred. Jo Beth's death need not have been so difficult. Had Jo Beth been in a hospice program, she would have had the advantage of having a physician that understood the needs of the terminally ill. Hospice nurses would have comforted her and helped her as she completed the work of dying. Her friend and daughters would have had the same support. She would not have been an obscure 38-year-old female with cancer of the breast. She would have been viewed as a valued human being with her needs and desires honored.

Hospice seeks to dispel the conspiracy of silence and avoidance. The philosophy of hospice is to view death as a natural part of life. Hospice nurses know that while cure may not be possible, peace and contentment are attainable. The entire interdisciplinary team seeks to assist the patient to attain a sense of peace and wholeness; to be physically, mentally, emotionally, and spiritually at peace.

HISTORICAL PERSPECTIVE

Hospice is a concept of care derived from medieval times. Hospices were first established by religious orders in Europe during the Middle Ages. Hospices were originally way stations for travelers and religious pilgrims where they could find food, lodging, and medical care on their journeys. Some provided care for the sick and the dying as well.

The modern hospice movement can be attributed largely to the work of one woman, Dame Cicely Saunders. Chase (1986) gave a vivid historical perspective of Cicely Saunder's life. In 1940, Saunders attended Nightingale Training School where she received her nursing education. As a nurse, she worked in the areas of gynecology and surgery, as well as with the mentally ill during World War II. After hurting her back, Saunders trained for a less physically demanding job as a "lady almoner," or medical social worker of that day. As an almoner she went to work in a hospital in England that specialized in caring for cancer patients. While working with cancer patients, she met David Tasma. Her relationship with Tasma would change her life and his.

Chase (1986) described Tasma as a 40-year-old Polish Jew who escaped from Poland to England during World War II. A refugee in a strange land with a different religion, he was truly a foreigner. In addition, he was diagnosed with cancer. Tasma was not ready to die. He wanted to come to terms with his life, to find peace and meaning. For this, Tasma needed more than good medical care, he needed a place to heal. Saunders was touched by Tasma's misfortune and devoted herself to helping him. Together, they searched for meaning to life and death. In the end, Tasma found the peace he was seeking and Saunders found that the dying have much to offer. Many of their talks centered on the need for a special place for those diagnosed with a terminal illness. A place was needed where the dying could receive the specialized care that would meet their unique needs. These discussions provided the seeds that would germinate into the development of St. Christopher's Hospice. At his death, Tasma left Saunders a small legacy. This legacy became the first donation to St. Christopher's (Chase, 1986).

After Tasma's death, Saunders, at the age of 33, decided to study medicine. Following her graduation from medical school, she focused on pain management. Saunders put her philosophy of caring for the dying into practice when St. Christopher's Hospice opened in June, 1967 in London, England. Saunders incorporated a number of innovative ideas into practice. These ideas included regulating medication based on the needs of the patient, allowing nurses discretion in the administration of pain medication, and giving medications orally instead of by injection. Her ideas were not always popular because they did not coincide with the ideas of the established medical profession. While skepticism prevailed, her success abounded. Her patients were alert and content and developed a sense of peace in the caring atmosphere provided at St. Christopher's (Stoddard, 1978).

In 1963, Dr. Saunders spoke about the hospice philosophy to a group of medical professionals, nurses, social workers, and clergy in New Haven, Connecticut. In 1974, Hospice, Inc. was established in Branford, Connecticut using as its model St.

Christopher's Hospice in London. Within the next decade, the hospice philosophy gained acceptance in the United States and eventually spread throughout the nation.

THE HOSPICE OF TODAY

Hospice services are one of the fastest growing segments of the health care industry. There are currently over 1800 hospice programs in the United States. Unlike hospitals, hospice programs strive to increase the length of stay of their patients. Patients referred within weeks or days of death are not able to reap the full benefits of the entire spectrum of hospice care. The more time patients spend in hospice care, the more the patient and family can benefit from the services provided. Patients enter hospice care when aggressive medical treatment is no longer an option, or when patients refuse aggressive medical treatment. Generally, only palliative, not curative, therapies are used.

Hospice stands out as a beacon of light to those suffering from terminal illness and families coping with anticipatory grief. Both the terminally ill patient and the family are actively engaged in the grieving process as they face the inevitability of death. This anticipatory grief can be overpowering if faced alone. Affiliation with a hospice program enables the terminally ill patient to have some measure of control over life. Feelings of control help the dying patient to have a more fulfilling and peaceful life as the day of death approaches. Special consideration is afforded to the family in the form of guidance, support, and encouragement. The interdisciplinary approach brings a variety of professionals together with one goal: to maximize the quality of life remaining for the patient and family.

A MODEL FOR UNDERSTANDING HOSPICE

The concept of hospice is one of holistic care and brings into focus four dimensions of support: physical, emotional, social, and spiritual. Welk (1991) characterized the concept of hospice utilizing interlocking circles (see figure 3.1). This model illustrates the four dimensions of support offered by hospice and the issues

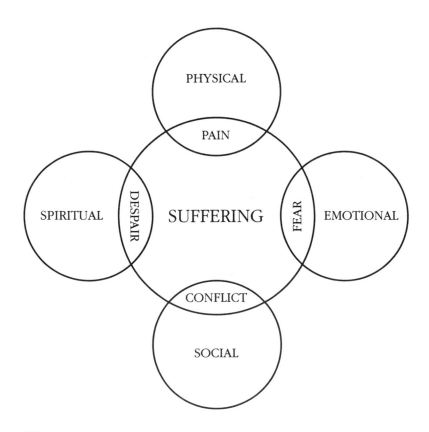

FIGURE 3.1

From an Educational Model for Explaining Hospice Services by J. A. Welk, 1991, *The American Journal of Hospice and Palliative Care*, Sept./Oct., pp. 14-17. Copyright 1991 by J. A. Welk. Reprinted by permission.

that must be faced as death becomes a reality. The center of Welk's model depicts suffering as the primary issue. An individual can be at peace only when suffering is alleviated. The goal of hospice is to alleviate suffering and achieve wholeness using the four basic dimensions of support.

Physical Dimension

The first dimension proposed by Welk is the physical dimension. Physical pain causes suffering. Unless physical pain is controlled, other dimensions cannot be fully addressed. Pain and suffering, however, are not always interchangeable, and a distinction must be made between the two. Suffering is more encompassing, affecting a person's entire being. Pain is more focused (Welk, 1991). An individual can experience no actual physical pain, yet be suffering immensely, as in the pain of watching a loved one die. Similarly, a patient may be in physical pain, yet not suffering. For example, an athlete engaged in the rough and vigorous activities of an important game may be so focused that she feels no pain, even when injured. Afterwards, she may have a multiplicity of aches and pains, yet not be suffering at all. She may in fact be exuberant. So pain does not always equate with suffering.

However, the issue of physical pain cannot be ignored since many hospice patients do suffer tremendous pain and discomfort. One major fear of the terminally ill patient and his family is the fear that the pain cannot be successfully managed outside the hospital setting. Therefore, a major focus of the hospice nurse is controlling physical pain. The patient and the family must be secure in the knowledge that pain management is an area where physicians and nurses working with hospice are truly experts. Hospice programs are extraordinarily successful in pain management. Once pain is controlled, that aspect of suffering is diminished and the patient is comforted. Although, as previously noted, successful management of physical pain does not necessarily alleviate suffering.

Emotional Dimension

The second interlocking circle depicted by Welk is the emotional dimension. Emotions are our feelings. The hospice patient is bombarded with various emotions, predominantly fear. Emotional suffering results in fear, with fear of death being the paramount fear. Death is an experience never faced before. One terminally ill patient stated, "I have never died before. I don't know how to do it. I don't know how it feels." Many patients are afraid that their families will be unable to cope with their death.

Terminally ill patients also do not want to die alone. Hospice patients do not die alone or in the hospital unless it is their choice. The hospice patient spends the last hours at home surrounded by family and friends in an atmosphere of love and acceptance. When patients acknowledge and accept their fears, trust evolves and suffering is reduced.

Social Dimension

The third dimension is the social dimension. No one lives in isolation. Relationships play a vital role in providing meaning and balance to our lives. According to Welk (1991), social suffering is expressed through conflict, most often conflict within relationships. The terminally ill patient needs to become reconciled with every individual, family member, or friend where there is significant conflict. Forgiveness and honesty are necessary to heal relationships and resolve conflict. Dying people must identify conflicts within relationships to restore balance and wholeness.

For some, the need to bid farewell to family and friends is important. This is observed in patients who, for no medical reason, continue to hang on to the threads of life until a long-awaited family member arrives. Shortly after the arrival, they die. Saying good-bye brings closure to relationships and peace to those at the end of their earthly lives.

Other concerns that affect the social dimension and may cause conflict are legal issues and financial matters. Many patients need to take care of unfinished business. Others who have always taken care of certain aspects of a relationship can feel no peace until that facet of the relationship is completed to their satisfaction. For example, the husband who has always taken care of his wife refuses to die until the repairs on her car are complete and the car is in good working order. The priority, however, in the social realm is to obtain reconciliation within relationships. Resolution of conflict will decrease social suffering and allow peace to follow (Welk, 1991).

Spiritual Dimension

The last interlocking circle described by Welk represents the spiritual aspect of hospice. Spiritual suffering causes despair.

Spirituality is often neglected until death approaches and denial is difficult. Welk believes this need is the most complex of the human needs. Spirituality is the method through which meaning and significance is given to life. It is how we define ourselves and transcends mere physical possessions. Spirituality is our search for who we are and why we are here. Without satisfactory answers, considerable suffering occurs, causing despair. Each individual meets the need for spirituality in her own way. For some, deep religious faith or a rich prayer life sustains them and gives meaning to life. For others, spirituality may be more subtle and spiritual peace may be sought in music, art, or nature. Igou (1984) felt that "helping the dying person to acknowledge his or her own spiritual nature can help give the remaining period of life its fullest meaning" (p. 158).

Hope is the most frequent word used to describe the essence of the spiritual realm (Welk, 1991). The interdisciplinary support offered by hospice increases hope. Hope reduces and sometimes relieves spiritual suffering. Through hope the future is faced with courage and strength.

The Holistic Aspect

Hospice acknowledges that patients are more than physical beings with physical needs. Spiritual, emotional, social, and physical needs become integrated to form the whole. These four dimensions represent the ongoing nature of the holistic care offered through hospice. In caring for the terminally ill, failure to address any one of these components results in suffering (Welk, 1991). The goal of hospice is to assist the patient and the family to reach a state of wholeness by alleviating (as much as possible) suffering in all four dimensions.

To diminish suffering requires immense effort and courage by the patient, the family, and all members of the health care team. Meeting the needs of the terminally ill requires specific skills and knowledge that are often lacking. The reluctance of nurses, physicians, and society to openly address the issues of death and dying contributes to the suffering of the terminally ill patient. Nurse-healers are able to address these issues and guide the patient toward wholeness.

HOLISTIC CARE

Managing the care of a dying patient requires many skills. Because of the complexity of care needed by the hospice patient, an interdisciplinary team composed of a variety of individuals, both professional and nonprofessional, is essential. This interdisciplinary team is composed of physicians, nurses, social workers, clergy, psychologists, home health aids, and volunteers. Although each member has certain expertise, there is an overlapping of the roles because each team member must be aware of needs that may arise in all areas. Needs may be simple, requiring intervention by only a few members of the team. Other patients and families may have complex needs that require the intervention of all of the interdisciplinary team. The interdisciplinary team meets regularly to problem solve, make decisions, and assure that care is coordinated (Downs, 1984).

The Role of the Nurse

The nurse most often serves as coordinator of care or case manager. The nurse has the theoretical background, knowledge, and technical proficiency to serve in the role of case manager (Downs, 1984). However, more than just skill and theoretical background are necessary. The nurse must become a healer. A willingness to share in the suffering and pain of the patient and the family is essential. Nurses often fear personal involve-ment because this brings them face to face with their own mortality. Hospice nurses must face death each day. They deal with the effects of pain, discouragement, and fear. Patients need the personal involvement of a nurse to guide them through a journey never faced before. The nurse-healer views nursing as a unique opportunity to form a close, meaningful relationship with another human being. Death brings on an openness and honesty between patients and nurses that other settings do not provide. Nurses become aware of many details about their patients' lives, loves, and losses. Family skeletons that have been hidden for years sometimes surface. The patient can often discuss his fear and uncertainty of death with the nurse more easily than with the family. Hospice nurses are rewarded by the opportunity to observe tangible results of their efforts, such as lessening of pain, calming of fears, easing of passage, and spiritual growth. Few nursing environments offer the nurse this unique opportunity (Cooke, 1992).

Principles of Pain Management

No discussion of hospice would be complete without addressing the management of pain, a central component of hospice care. Pain control is very important. Effective management of pain is possible in over 95% of all patients (Johanson, 1993). The medication that has proven most effective is morphine sulfate. Nurses are often reluctant to give adequate dosages of morphine for fear of complications. Patients and their families can suffer needlessly when pain is not managed appropriately. Kay's experience illustrates one nurse's lack of understanding of the use of morphine for the relief of pain.

Kay's Experience with Death

Kay's mother had been ill for several years. The cancer that had begun in her colon had now spread to her liver. Although she was only 15 years old, Kay had learned to care for her mother and had done so throughout her illness. Now her mother's long battle was almost over and she was approaching the point of death. Kay's mother was weak and restless. Her breathing was shallow and labored. Although semicomatose, she was moaning with pain. The nurse came into the room after Kay pushed the call light, but his face became anxious when Kay requested something to ease her mother's pain and discomfort. The nurse explained to Kay that he could give her mother the morphine sulfate that was ordered by the doctor. But while the morphine would ease the pain, it would almost certainly depress her respirations to the point of death. Kay emphatically said that she wanted her mother's comfort above all else. Morphine was given. Kay sat close to the bedside and held her mother's hand. Surprisingly, after about 20 minutes, her mother's breathing improved and her pain was less. Her pain-ridden face relaxed and, miraculously, her respirations were normal. The nurse came quickly after Kay's call and was amazed at the sight of his patient so much improved. The remainder of the night was spent quietly. Kay's mother died peacefully the next morning.

In many ways, this was a brave nurse. He risked what he thought might cause death to ease the pain and suffering of his patient. His compassion outweighed his fear. The misconception that morphine significantly depresses respirations when given for severe pain has been perpetuated for many years. Today, we know that when morphine is used to control severe pain, it does not produce the respiratory depressant effect that was once thought to be so significant (Johanson, 1993). Although the incident mentioned above occurred several years ago, many nurses today still do not understand the use of morphine for severe pain. Johanson (1993) identified the principles involved in administering opiates for pain relief (see table 3.1).

Assisting the Hospice Patient

The goal for hospice is to assist the patient to live life to the fullest and to find a sense of purpose and meaning. Unfortunately, not every patient can achieve total peace and serenity. Most often death is met with the same attitudes and coping mechanisms used throughout life. However, there is a unique opportunity for growth with anticipatory death. There is time to prepare, say good-bye, become reconciled with estranged loved ones, and discuss the future without the loved one.

Helping the terminally ill progress through the process of grief is not an easy task. Grieving is hard work, whether it is for self or for a loved one. When someone knows that he has only a limited time to live, he is forced to come to terms with his life. Successes as well as failures must be faced. In life, there is always the feeling that some day I will resolve this issue or someday I will reach that goal. However, time is not a commodity that the dying have to spare. Issues that have long been postponed must be faced. The

1. The drug of choice for severe pain in terminal care is oral morphine sulphate.

2. Morphine is versatile, safe and effective for almost all severe cancer pain.

3. Pain from a constant source must be anticipated and treated with regular dosing *before* the return of pain.

4. The most important factor in determining proper dosage is a patient's resultant sense of mental well-being.

5. Excess sedation or euphoria is *not* a goal of palliative therapy.

6. Pain is an opiate antagonist (It counteracts the sedative and respiratory depressant effects of morphine).

7. All opiates cause dependence but people in severe pain do not develop addictive psychological behavior.

8. The need to steadily increase dosage for reasons of tolerance has not proven to be a significant problem.

9. The use of morphine does not shorten a patient's life.

10. Morphine exists to be given — not withheld.

TABLE 3.1   Principles of Pain Management

From *Physicians Handbook of Symptom Relief in Terminal Care* (4th ed.) (p. 4.6) by G.A. Johanson. Sonoma County Academic Foundation for Excellence in Medicine. Copyright 1993. Adapted by permission.

anguish felt by family members when watching a loved one suffer cannot be ignored. With anticipatory death, this anguish can last for months before death and linger afterwards for several years.

Hope

Hope is an important issue. Many are concerned with giving false hope. Others are concerned with taking away all hope. Because the future is never completely predictable, the truth can be presented with an element of hope. If the hospice patient can accept the fact that cure may not be possible, the spiritual part of the person can take over. Spirituality can then activate the healing process. Goals become to restore harmony and balance in life and to be at peace with death.

Hope is necessary for all patients. Hope is strengthened by the patient's confidence and trust in the nurse. Trust and confidence are enhanced if the nurse is sincere, compassionate, and accessible. The nurse can never say, "I've done all I can do." This is a fallacy that must not be perpetuated because something can always be done. Nurses may sit beside the bed, hold the patient's hand, give a back rub, or place a cool cloth to the face. The nurse's presence confirms the nurse's compassion and gives comfort. Nurses must foster hope to help the patient to reach the highest level of peace possible and to continue to live to the fullest.

> Hope, like a gleaming taper's light,
> Adorns and cheers our way;
> and still as darker groweth the night,
> Emits a brighter day.
>   Oliver Goldsmith

The Search for Meaning

The search for meaning to life becomes a priority for many. The search for meaning is important because a positive meaning can make life worthwhile, allowing death to go on with peacefulness and dignity. If no positive meaning can be found, a person's life is viewed as a failure. Death, then, becomes the ultimate failure. Despair prevails. To prevent this fatalistic view, the nurse must help the patient in her search for meaning. This is done by actively listening as the patient speaks, gently focusing on important areas identified by the patient, and providing positive guidance and direction. Reminiscing is one way to begin this search. The conclusions reached in the search for meaning are the patient's insights, not the nurse's. David's search for meaning is depicted in the following vignette.

David's Search for Meaning

David's search for meaning was more dramatic than most. David was a 78-year-old retired English professor. Much of his life was spent engrossed in his work. However, after a bitter battle with lung cancer, he was a hospice patient in a home setting. David's anger and resentment posed problems in communication for the nurse, but she persisted. After several weeks of daily visits with David, he became less angry and more verbal. The nurse began by asking him about his work and as he reminisced, he appeared more discontented than angry. There was always the undertone of bitterness. One day David appeared unusually quiet. The nurse gently questioned his behavior. Without warning, David began to sob and revealed an incident over 20 years ago. A young woman had become pregnant by David, but he had refused to marry her, totally rejecting both the mother and the unborn child. The young woman left and he had never heard from her again. The nurse listened to David's tearful story, talked to several individuals, and within two weeks David's lost child was found. His daughter was a graduate student in David's own field of study. Remarkably, she wanted to meet David. After a shaky first meeting, David and his daughter reconciled. David was able to visit with his daughter. David told his nurse, "At last, I know what my life was truly about."

David died a peaceful death. He was no longer bitter, having found reconciliation and meaning. At times, as with David, the nurse is the one who sees the need and initiates (with the patient's permission) reconciliation.

The Family

In most hospice programs, the family members are the caretakers. One specific family member usually has the major responsibility, with other family members helping. Taking care of one who is dying is difficult and demands tremendous energy and courage. Many caregivers sacrifice their own health in order to care for their loved one. Guilt is a normal response in those who are not able to participate in the care. However, even those who give continuous 24-hour-a-day care are often critical of themselves. This critical attitude contributes to feelings of guilt. The nurse must emphasize that this type of guilt is normal and natural, but unnecessary.

It is essential that caretakers take time away from the loved one for themselves. Time spent away from the pressures of caring for the loved one is important for effective coping. A quiet time alone, a walk by the ocean, music, a massage, or exercise may be avenues of momentary escape for the caregiver.

Caregivers often do not know what to do or say. They focus on the physical care, neglecting the psychosocial facets of care. Caregivers need to be taught what to do and what to say. Table 3.2 provides suggestions for the nurse to give caregivers to help them in knowing what they can do for themselves and their loved one.

The Importance of Communication

Psychological needs can best be met through communication. Talking with the patient is perhaps the most significant thing any-

---

1. Expect emotions to fluctuate. Anger, sadness, depression, frustration, laughter and tears may be experienced on a daily basis. Accept these emotions. They are normal.

2. Any of the psychological and physical symptoms associated with grief may be experienced by the caretaker prior to the death as well as afterwards.

3. Give your full attention to your loved one. If need be, say, "I love you," "I'm sorry," "Good-bye," "I forgive you."

4. Be affectionate. Touch. Hold hands, kiss, and/or embrace.

5. Reminisce. Talk about the loved one's accomplishments, special memories, joys, heartaches.

6. Ask about the loved one's feelings on funeral arrangements, how he would like to be remembered, special songs or poems.

7. Talk and actively listen to what is being said.

8. Give the loved one permission to die.

9. Reconcile any differences you have with your loved one.

10. Engage in pleasurable activities together.

TABLE 3.2   *Guidelines for Caregivers*

one can do. Too often people are afraid to talk. They do not know what to say. They are afraid of saying the wrong thing.

Caregivers and family must know the importance of listening and talking, of saying, "I love you," "I'm sorry," and, when appropriate, "Good-bye." Failure to express these feelings can be a source of deep regret to families and friends. It is also important to be affectionate through touching or hugging. People often have difficulty touching the patient. They seem to be afraid of "catching" the disease or of hurting a fragile body. Gently touching the skin can be very calming.

Surprisingly, discussions of the future can also be therapeutic. Talking about the future can relieve anxieties the dying person has about another family member. A dying mother can be comforted knowing the future plans of a teenage son or daughter.

Sometimes discussions of the future provide an opportunity to bring up funeral arrangements. Families need to know if the patient has any desire to participate in plans for the funeral or any particular wishes or requests. The family, however, must be open to cues that show these matters are not significant to the patient. Some patients are eager to address the topic of their funeral. They may express desires for special songs to be sung at the funeral, those they wish to officiate, or where they want to be buried. Some may want to plan the entire service, even to selecting the casket. A young woman, fearing death was near, and without anyone's knowledge, planned her entire funeral. She chose the casket, the clothing she would wear, and the time of day for the funeral. She stated she did not want her family to go through the pain of making these difficult choices. Another woman wanted her funeral procession to go straight down May Street in Oklahoma City. She stated, "I have been stopped in traffic going down that street for years, and just once I would like traffic to stop for me."

Communication also allows expressions of how the loved one will be remembered or how he influenced another's life. The following statements provide comfort: "Whenever I see a yellow rose, I'll remember our anniversary and all the wonderful times we've had together," or "I'll never forget that week we spent in Paris. It was the greatest time of my life," or "Remember that camping trip at Thanksgiving? That was the best camping trip I have ever been on."

Giving the loved one permission to die is often the most difficult thing for family and friends to do. Statements giving permission to die include: "I love you with all my heart, but I'll be OK," or "Life will be fuller because you have been a part of it," or simply saying, "Mama, it's OK! I'll be all right. You can go if you want to." These statements are difficult to say, but necessary for a peaceful death.

The patient, besides feeling the love and support of family members, must feel that her loved ones will be able to survive the death. If peace is attained, then death can be faced with a measure of anticipation and contentment.

Hospice Care: Not for Everyone

The focus of hospice care is on palliative, not curative care. This type of focus is not suitable for all dying patients or their families. Some families cannot easily let go of their loved one and need the heroic measures provided by doctors and nurses in an acute care setting. These families want every technological means possible used to prolong the life of their loved one in the hope that a cure will be found. They may view hospice care as giving up or indicative of not caring enough.

Some families cannot provide the home care their loved one needs. Other families may want the security of the hospital where health care professionals can provide the daily hands-on care so necessary for the dying patient. Still others may choose hospice care, but when their loved one begins to actively die, they may be unable to resist the temptation to dial 911.

Despite the reason, hospice care is not a workable option for all families. The nurse must respect the decision of the patient and the family. Whatever the choice, support and guidance are needed in any setting where death occurs and families are grieving.

BEREAVEMENT CARE

Hospice care does not end with the death of the patient. Bereavement follow-up is essential to help the family in completing the grieving process. Research by Ransford and Smith (1991) suggested that grief resolution is significantly higher after one year in families whose loved one received hospice care than in the bereaved of those who died in a hospital setting.

Despite the amount of preparation, no one is ever totally ready to part with a loved one. A family can become so caught up in the caregiving aspect that death comes as a surprise. On the other hand, a family can feel tremendous relief from the pain and suffering. Feelings of relief are often followed by guilt. Families need assistance in the satisfactory resolution of grief. If hospice services have been used to the fullest prior to the death, the grieving process may be less intense and less stressful. Hospice can provide avenues for the family to be reconciled, to say their good-byes, and to find meaning. These families may need minimal support. Other families may be less prepared and need more guidance.

Hospice nurses play a significant role in guiding and supporting grieving families. The hospice nurse is often the one who the family calls first when death occurs, the one who pronounces death, and the one who stays with the family as the realization that death is a reality occurs. Hospice nurses like Esperanza in the following vignette can facilitate the healing process in the initial stages of grief.

Esperanza's Story

Esperanza, a hospice nurse, had been caring for Mr. Garcia, a kindly 74-year-old gentleman, for several weeks. The family was close and Mr. Garcia had devoted much of his time to his grandchildren. He was father to 10 children and grandfather to 18 youngsters ranging from 6 to 14 years of age. At 6:30 P.M., Esperanza received a call from Mr. Garcia's family. They were frightened. His breathing was diminishing and he was growing weaker. Esperanza told the family she would come immediately. When she arrived at the Garcia home, Esperanza found that Mr. Garcia had died. The grandchildren were sobbing. Their grief was great. Esperanza quietly took care of her responsibilities concerning Mr. Garcia. She then turned her attention to the grandchildren. Esperanza quickly gathered the 12 or so children around her and quieted them with her soft words of kindness. She asked that each child whisper in her ear one cherished memory about their grandpa. Timidly the first child came and whispered into her ear. Esperanza smiled and quietly shared with the grieving family the special time Grandpa took little John fishing for the first time. Each child came to whisper to Esperanza that special memory of Grandpa. Afterwards, the house was quiet with the family members remembering the special place this man had in their hearts.

Esperanza initiated healing by encouraging positive reminiscing. Hospice nurse-healers are in a special position to initiate and facilitate healing and growth within families.

Most hospice programs have bereavement follow-up programs to help mourners in reaching these goals. The nurse attends the funeral, visits with the family, provides individual support, and organizes support groups and memorial services.

Bereavement programs may be formal or informal. Formal groups meet regularly for five or six weeks. Grief is a subject most are unfamiliar with and the topic is often taboo in our society. Because of this unfamiliarity, bereavement programs must focus on what constitutes the grieving process. Feelings to expect, how to progress through grief, and how to look to the future with hope are also areas of focus. While the entire grieving process may take many years, most of the grief work described by Lindemann in chapter 1 can be done in two to three years. Hospice can facilitate grieving and assist the family in gaining a sense of meaning within a shorter period.

Hospice care is extended to the family after death has occurred. Bereavement care is an integral part of the services offered. Grieving often begins before death (anticipatory grief) and extends for several months to several years afterward. The physical, spiritual, emotional, and social well-being of the family is considered before the death and afterward. Bereavement follow-up offers counseling, support groups, and memorial services to help the resolution of grief. Hospice cannot totally eliminate the pain and suffering of grief, but it can assist and support the bereaved through this process.

SUMMARY

Hospice care begins with admission to the program, continues throughout illness and death, and lasts an indefinite time afterward as the family continues through the grieving process. This concept of care began in medieval times as places that served as sanctuaries for travelers, the ill, and the homeless. The modern day concept of hospice is a place where the terminally ill patient and the family can find solace in a society where even the words *death, dying,* and *terminally ill* are often shunned.

The entire hospice team is interdisciplinary, with nurses at the hub, managing the holistic care. Special attention is given to both the family and the patient and the complex problems that emerge as death approaches.

Human beings are not one-dimensional. Spiritual, social, physical, and emotional dimensions all affect the individual. Hospice addresses needs in each dimension to decrease the pain and suffering and guide the patient to peace. The holistic approach recognizes that if needs in one area are not met, then all areas suffer.

Patients facing death grieve, and need time and nurturing to heal. Healing is manifested as the suffering of each dimension is eliminated or alleviated and life's meaning is validated. The holistic care offered in hospice is vital for the patient and the family to reach the peace and contentment necessary for healing.

REFLECTIONS

1. How has your understanding and appreciation of hospice changed?

2. Can you talk openly and honestly with a terminally ill patient? Do you either consciously or unconsciously avoid contact with those who are terminally ill?

3. What are your feelings concerning the administration of morphine to patients in severe pain?

4. How can you use the holistic philosophy of care in your own practice?

References

Chase, D. (1986). *Dying at home with hospice.* St. Louis: C. V. Mosby Company.

Cooke, M. (1992, January/February). The challenge of hospice nursing in the 90's. *The American Journal of Palliative Care,* pp. 34–37.

Downs, M. (1984). The hospice team. In S. H. Schraff (Ed.), *Hospice: The nursing perspective* (pp. 47–57). New York: National League for Nursing.

Igou, I. (1984). Current issues and future directions. In S. H. Schraff (Ed.), *Hospice: The nursing perspective* (pp. 153–167). New York: National League for Nursing.

Johanson, G. A. (1993). *Physician's handbook of symptom relief in terminal care* (4th ed.). Santa Rosa, CA: Sonoma County Academic Foundation for Excellence in Medicine.

Ransford, H., & Smith, M. (1991). Grief resolution among the bereaved in hospice and hospital wards. *Social Science Medicine, 32*(3), 295–304.

Stoddard, S. (1978). *The hospice movement: A better way of caring for the dying.* Briar Cliff Manor, NY: Stein and Day Publishers.

Welk, J. A. (1991, September/October). An educational model for explaining hospice services. *The American Journal of Hospice and Palliative Care,* pp. 14–17.

SURVIVING THE LOSS OF A LOVED ONE

4

Sally S. Roach

*When you are sorrowful, look again in your heart,
and you shall see that in truth you are weeping for
that which has been your delight.*

Kahlil Gibran, *The Prophet*

INTRODUCTION

Our lives are shaped by our relationships with those around us. These relationships help define who we are, give meaning to life, and provide social structure. "What I am at any given moment in the process of my becoming a person will be determined by my relationships with those who love me or refuse to love me, with those I love or refuse to love" (Powell, 1969, p. 43). Relationships with children, parents, a spouse, or a partner all play a significant role in defining who we are. When death destroys any of these relationships, we not only mourn the loved one, but the loss of the relationship as well. This chapter explores the grief experienced with the loss of each of the preceding relationships. The grief experienced is proportional to the significance that the relationship had in sustaining and balancing the individual's life. The greater the emotional attachment, the greater the number of needs met by the relationship, and the greater the loss. Bugen (1977) found that the loss of central relationships produced more severe reactions than the loss of ancillary relationships. Central relationships are not bound by formal or legal ties, but can include lovers, soul mates, special friends, even mentors. They can be relationships of the same sex or of different sexes. While the term *spouse* is used to denote one type of central relationship, the reader should be aware that loss of any central relationship can elicit similar feelings and intense grief.

Surviving the loss of a loved one is a difficult experience. To complicate the process, most people are unprepared for the pain and intensity of feelings that take control of their lives. Death often occurs without warning, and even with anticipatory grief, individuals are never really prepared for the finality of death. The survivors are stranded in a sea of emotions that ebb and flow as the tides.

Additionally, the survivors may lose a particular lifestyle or social role. For example, a widow of a busy executive may find herself excluded from social functions or dinner parties that she once attended with her husband. Or a young couple who lose a child may find themselves uncomfortable with parents of their child's friends. The bereaved parents may resent others who have healthy children.

Loss of future dreams or expectations may be a part of the grief experience. The long-awaited retirement will never be realized, the special trip will never be taken, the anticipated promotion will never occur, or the joy of the child's accomplishments will never be experienced. Future expectations in these areas must be modified and sometimes changed altogether. Death, then, is not simply a loss of a special relationship, but the loss of an idealized vision of the future.

THE DEATH OF A CHILD

The relationship between mother and child is special and begins before the actual birth of the infant. The mother begins to feel a special closeness and attachment to the infant early as changes occur in her body with pregnancy. At birth, or before, the father begins to feel a certain closeness as well. After the birth, the child becomes an integral part of their lives. The child grows from infancy to childhood, then adolescence, and finally to adulthood. Each developmental stage harbors its own unique love and promotes dreams for the future.

Parents who lose children will quickly attest to the fact that the most overwhelming and devastating loss is the loss of a child. A child represents a part of the parents, a source of joy for the present, and a portion of the parents' contribution to future generations. When a child dies, the loss is twofold: (1) loss of that special part of the parents and (2) loss of a portion of the parents' hopes and dreams for the future.

The death of a child in our society is usually so unexpected that it often seems unreal or impossible. The death is often viewed as a failure on the part of the parents, the fault of careless medical personnel, or as an abandonment by God. "How could God allow such a great atrocity as this to happen?"

The death of a child at any age is difficult and grief is profound. When adulthood is reached, the parents still feel a strong attachment, but the feelings are usually less intense (Raphael, 1983). However, when a child dies, no matter the age, a door to the future is closed and a vision of that child's contribution to the future is lost forever.

The Death of an Infant

The loss of an infant touches the very essence of our being. This little life is totally dependent on us for survival. Our sense of this responsibility is so profound that the loss of one so totally defenseless can cause immense grief. Characteristics seen in various types of death in infancy are summarized in table 4.1.

Although stillbirth, miscarriage, and neonatal death are somewhat different, a study by Peppers and Knapp (1980) found no significant differences in the intensity of the grief experienced.

Interventions of the Nurse-Healer

The nurse as a healer plays a vital role in the resolution of grief for the parents. The nurse is often the caregiver that has the most

Death	Characteristics
Miscarriage and Stillbirth	Parents, especially the mother, may have feelings of intense sadness, anger or guilt.
	The death is often inadequately recognized by others, especially if the loss occurs in early weeks of pregnancy.
	The death may be considered a personal failure.
	Parents may dwell on details, designating blame to themselves or others.
	Grief from previous miscarriages may be relived.
	Anticipatory grief may occur if the condition of the infant is known early.
	Ambivalence experienced in early pregnancy may increase grief.
	Hopes for the future must be modified or changed.
	Despair may peak when the parents must leave the hospital without the baby.
Neonatal Death	Feelings are similar to stillbirth.
	Parents have had the time to form a bond with the infant, intensifying the grief.
	Grief may be intense by both parents.
Sudden Infant Death Syndrome (SIDS)	Death is unexplainable and totally unexpected.
	Pain is increased by lack of knowledge and misinformation.
	Parental bonding is complete.
	Death is silent, no signs of distress.
	Guilt may be present.
	Police may investigate, adding to the guilt.
	Grief is acute since there is no time to prepare.
	Parents, especially the mother, may be preoccupied with the details of the death.
Abortion	Shame, secrecy, and guilt may accompany grief.
	Highly ambivalent feelings may be present.
	Little support or comfort is offered by others.
	Feelings of relief are expected, but despair and depression may surface.
	No guilt may be felt, especially if the woman did not want a child.

TABLE 4.1   Death of a Child in Infancy

communication with the parents. Care must be taken to offer support and to assist in validation of the loss. With the loss of a child, all areas of life career out of balance. The wound is deep and severe. Time is needed for healing. Parents who lose a child through stillbirth or miscarriage are often not given permission to grieve. They are expected to move through grief with such a rapid progression that the grief is denied or muffled (Hutti, 1988). Cliches such as, "You can have another baby," "The fetus was probably defective anyway," or "It must be God's will," will suppress grieving and isolate parents from the healer.

Nurse-healers must realize that even in planned pregnancies some reservation is present. Particularly in early pregnancy, parents vacillate in varying degrees about assuming the parental role. Even when the baby is planned and anxiously awaited, some unspoken doubts occur. Then if death occurs, parents feel guilt and may view the loss as a punishment. The healer's reassurance is necessary. Giving verbal permission to grieve promotes healing (Hutti, 1988).

The family and other members of the support system need to understand the parental need to relive and discuss the loss fo as long as a year or more after the death has occurred (Hut 1988). Feelings of isolation and depression intensify when t' need to verbalize thoughts and feelings is not recognized as p of healing.

Nurse-healers must also teach families the normal respo of grief. Intense feelings of loss are common for bereaved ents and reassurance that these intense feelings are a norma of the grieving process is important. Everyone journeys th grief at their own pace. Parents must be made aware t' some the journey is long and difficult. Others are able t more easily through the healing process. Awareness of thi the parents to accept their own particular passage thro and helps family members to be more understanding wh ing is more difficult.

In order to validate the loss, parents should be ; see and hold their child after death if they choose Before viewing the child, the parents should be prep description of the looks of the child, including any Even if the baby is abnormal, the parents' vision o' appearance is usually worse than the actual appe

1988). After seeing the infant, parents tend to focus on the positive attributes rather than on any negative qualities (Kellner, Donnelly, & Gould, 1984). Nurse-healers can ease this process by identifying positive features such as hair of the same color as the parents, the shape of the hands or the face, or the beauty that is present in every creation. Tangible mementos such as footprints, identification bracelets, or a lock of hair may be comforting to parents (Hutti, 1988).

Effects of a Child's Death on the Husband/Wife Relationship

The death of a child causes a great deal of tension in the marital relationship. The tension can be so stressful that parents may contemplate separation or divorce. Relationships that were strong before the death weather the storms of grief better than relationships that were rocky before the child's death. After the death, parents may no longer have the emotional energy or inclination to continue the struggle necessary to save the marriage (Klass, 1986–87).

Schwab (1992) examined the effects of a child's death on the parents' marital relationship. His study identified the following themes: husband's concern about wife's grief, wife's anger over husband's reluctance to share grief, problems communicating effectively, decrease in sexual intimacy, and generalized irritability. Schwab's (1992) findings are summarized in the following sections.

Husband's Concern About His Wife's Grief   The grief experienced by most women is very intense. The husband often feels totally helpless to assist the wife in overcoming her grief. Whatever he does seems to be wrong. In an effort not to add to the wife's grief, the husband may withdraw to grieve alone.

Wife's Anger Over Husband's Reluctance to Share Grief Ironically, the husband's reluctance to share grief may be caused by his desire to decrease his wife's pain. Some men, however, are not able to grieve openly. These men release feelings through action. Immersing themselves in work, starting a big project, or becoming involved in a sport are ways in which many men deal

with grief. Additionally, husbands often feel they must remain "strong" for the wife and other family members. They tend to avoid discussing the loss and allow themselves to grieve only when alone. This reluctance to share grief angers the wife who feels that her husband does not care or that she loved the child more and her suffering is greater.

Problems Communicating Effectively   The expression of grief is completely individual in nature. Some grieve openly. They weep and freely discuss the death. Others are deeply distressed but unable to verbalize feelings. Or, out of the desire not to increase the pain or upset the spouse, each partner may withdraw and communicate only superficially. Genuine communication ceases. True thoughts and feelings are not discussed on a meaningful level, but are hidden from the other.

Decrease in Sexual Intimacy   Most people have a decrease in sexual desire after a significant loss. Men may use sexual intimacy as a means of comfort. Women experience a decrease in sexual desire for much longer periods of time. As a result, a grieving woman often views sexual advances from her husband with extreme distaste and may reject her husband altogether.

Generalized Irritability   Each spouse experiences greater irritability and less tolerance toward the other. Past conflicts may resurface causing additional stress within the marital relationship.

Helping Parents to Heal

The nurse-healer can more effectively guide the griever if the themes identified by Schwab are understood and used to provide insight for the griever. However, the nurse should avoid stereotyping any reaction to loss. The themes identified by Schwab maybe reversed. That is, men can express grief the same way as women and expressions of grief may be similar in both sexes. Attention is focused on letting the spouses know that whatever responses they experience are normal within the context of grief. Emphasis is placed on the fact that there is no right way to grieve. When reactions are accepted as normal, the path is open for healing. The nurse-healer can then teach the couple more effective communication techniques and encourage them to work together to heal the wounds of the loss. In this way, the nurse can not only assist in healing the wounds of grief, but perhaps begin to heal wounds within the relationship as well.

Healing the wounds after the loss of a child occurs very slowly and requires much patience on the part of both the nurse and the parents. Their lives will never be the same again. Hopes and dreams of the future involving the child must be relinquished. It may take several years before any type of normalcy is restored in everyday living. Parents need nurturing through this difficult period. They need to be allowed to verbalize their feelings and be reassured that ultimately healing will occur.

THE DEATH OF A LIFE PARTNER

The marriage relationship is very complex. There are various levels of closeness in a marital relationship which lead to different responses if loss occurs. Raphael (1983) discussed two different types of closeness in marriage and the significance of loss in each. Most relationships fall somewhere in the spectrum between the two extremes that follow.

The first type of marital relationship occurs where each partner has a distinct and relatively separate lifestyle with minimal closeness. Sharing is predominantly superficial and may focus on family activities. In this type of relationship, the wife has her own friends, social life, and quite possibly, a career. She receives gratification and meaning in her life through these external activities rather than from the marriage itself. The husband, likewise, has his own circle of friends from whom he receives support and recreation. Interaction is minimal. As Raphael (1983) pointed out, the loss of a spouse in this type of relationship is significant, but it will elicit fewer grief responses than a relationship where the marriage takes precedence.

In the second type of marital relationship, the marriage itself is the focus of the relationship. The social life of the couple is shared completely. There is a strong commitment to family life. The couple regards communication, the expression of feelings, and the sharing of common values as very important. Sexuality and closeness play a vital role. Loss of a spouse in this type of relationship is extremely stressful and causes profound grief because so much of the spouses' lives are intertwined (Raphael, 1983).

For most couples, marriage was more than a superficial relationship. Marriage was described by Lightner and Hathaway (1990) as providing a companion; a friend; a lover; a helpmate; someone to share burdens, pleasures, decisions, and details of daily life. This intimate type of marriage provides structure and stability for each partner's life and helps define who they are. To lose a spouse in this type of relationship may mean losing a part of one's identity (Raphael, 1983). With death, the chief source of support is gone and the loss can be totally devastating.

THE DEATH OF A PARENT

The death of a parent can be particularly devastating even to adult children. Parents are a major link to the past and an anchor amid the turmoil of life in the present. In positive parent/child relationships, parents are the ones who always express love no matter what happens. They are the ones who can be called at any time, day or night, for a word of encouragement, a listening ear, or simply a friendly chat when one is lonely. The relationship with one's parents covers the longest time frame and perhaps is the one in which the most unconditional love is received. Jan, a wife, a mother, and a grandmother expresses the unconditional love of her own mother, who is long deceased, and the longing she still has for her.

A Mother's Love

My mother died over 30 years ago when I was a mere 16 years old. At the time, I loved her more than anything else in the world. I was crushed at her death and grieved for several years. Mostly I grieved alone, because I had no siblings with which to reminisce and my dad was immersed in his own grief. When I married, my husband had never known my mother and, of course, neither would my children. Over the last 30 years, my life has been rich and full. Basically every need that I have had has been met. There is, however, one exception. At times, I still very desperately need my mother. While my grief has long been resolved, this need for her is very real. I need her advice, her wisdom, her love. At times I awaken in the night with a deep longing for her. I want my mother to know my children, my husband, my accomplishments. No one has ever loved me so unconditionally, so purely, so totally nonjudgmentally as my mother. I wish I could simply have her near me again to comfort me with her presence and be a part of my life. I guess you never outgrow the need for your mother.

Jan's feelings are not unusual. The need for the love and support of a parent never fades. A study by Scharlach (1991) revealed that for as long as 5 years after the death of a parent many adult children still become upset and cry when thinking about the deceased parent. In addition, they still miss the parent a great deal. Scharlach (1991) also found that children who have a strong need for parental approval experience more distress.

Conflictual Relationships

Unresolved conflicts between parents and children can surface with the death of a parent. Children instinctively want to love their parents. However, issues arise within relationships that cause conflict and feelings of ambivalence. Ambivalence complicates the grieving process. Facing dissension and problems within relationships can cause deep-seated emotions to surface. When past conflicts surface, they must be dealt with before grief can continue and resolution occur. The nurse-healer can help the griever to view conflicts realistically. The cause of the dissension must then be examined and forgiveness must occur. Sometimes this requires forgiveness of self. At other times, as in the situation with George, forgiveness of the deceased is necessary. Only after forgiveness can grief continue.

Forgiving Dad

When George heard the news of his dad's death all he could feel was anger. For 42 years, George had been trying to gain his father's love and approval. To the outside world, George's dad was a "good old boy." To the three boys in the family, he was a man to be feared. His uncontrollable outbursts of temper were invariably aimed at one of them. George spent all of his life trying to gain his father's approval and love. He wanted desperately to have a good relationship with his dad. Now with his dad's death this desired relationship was impossible. As long as his father was alive, there was hope for reconciliation. Fortunately, George was able to obtain the counseling he needed. Through a bereavement support group, George was able to work through his feelings of anger and guilt. He was able, with time, to forgive his father and move through the grieving process.

George was fortunate to be able to use the death of his father to resolve a conflict within the relationship. Not everyone who has endured a conflictual relationship will be able to identify the root of the conflict, work through the emotional turmoil, and forgive themselves or the deceased.

For others, the death of a parent who was very controlling or overly critical can be almost liberating. For the first time, the adult child can make choices without the fear of criticism or follow a path of her own choosing without guilt.

THE DEATH OF A SIBLING

The death of a sibling is often one of those losses considered by society not to be as severe as other losses. The loss of a mother, a father, a spouse, or a child is most often considered to be of major significance. Society expects losses of this magnitude to elicit grief and the mourner has societal permission to grieve fully. After the loss of a sibling, however, society may not be so compassionate. Societal permission to grieve is limited. This is unfortunate since the relationship between siblings may be very strong even to the point of mimicking the parent-child relationship. A brother or a sister may serve as a protector, role model, or close friend. At other times, the relationship between siblings may be plagued with conflict. Conflictual relationships between siblings may complicate or delay grief.

Nurse-healers must be aware of the distress experienced at the loss of a sibling. Acknowledging the need to grieve and encouraging the expression of feelings will affirm the grief and assist in restoring balance.

EMOTIONAL ASPECTS OF GRIEF

It hurts to lose a loved one. The grief felt is a normal human response to loss. The emotions experienced are common to all humanity, male or female, young or old. The intensity to which these emotions are experienced and expressed vary.

Emotions are our feelings and the expression of those feelings. They arise from internal and external responses to life events. As the griever proceeds through the grieving process, many emotions surface. A few of the most prevalent emotions are anger, depression, loneliness, and guilt. The survivor is challenged to recognize and express, not suppress these emotions.

Anger

Anger is one of the most powerful emotions experienced and can range from mild irritation to rage. Anger is an expression of frustration over the lack of control over a situation. The mourner feels a sense of fury at being deserted by the loved one. The anger may be totally uncharacteristic of the mourner, adding stress upon stress. Fear of going crazy or losing it all may cause the mourner to withdraw or become depressed.

Expressions of Anger

The mourner realizes that it is impractical to be angry at the deceased, so that anger is displaced to anyone within close proximity. Doctors, nurses, friends, and other relatives are all vulnerable. Anger is expressed at nurses for not taking better care of the loved one, at God for permitting death, at friends for not expressing the right thought, or at other relatives for any perceived indiscretion, no matter how minor. Expressions of anger are portrayed in the following examples.

Anger at the Physician "Why didn't he take better care of Javier? Surely there was something more he could do. New techniques, new medications are discovered every day. Why wasn't the doctor aware of these new developments that could have possibly saved Javier's life? I was incensed at the doctor's lack of compassion, at the pain Javier was forced to endure. I know more could have been done."

Anger at the Deceased "Why did John have to die? Just when we were making plans for retirement. I was so angry at him for leaving me. We were going to take that vacation to Alaska that we always talked about, but never had time to take. Now I'm all alone. Who could enjoy a vacation alone? Just like John to leave me at the end of life with no life at all to look forward to. How could he do that to me?"

Anger at Friends "I can hardly stand it when Jane talks about how her husband, now retired, is always in her way. She says that he is always underfoot, never giving her any time alone. One day I couldn't stand it any more and said, "Why don't you try sleeping each night in a bed alone or sitting down to a meal with no one to share it with day after day? I would welcome someone in my house just to be nearby."

Anger at God "Why did God do this to my little Megan? A god who truly cares would never punish a helpless little child with the pain that Megan had to endure. I have such mixed feelings. Anger at God for allowing this to happen. Anger at myself for blaming God."

Anger at Relatives "I was so irritable with my children. Everything they did annoyed me. The constant nagging for something to eat, to watch TV, or for me to play with them. Usually, I have so much patience. Now I have none. It seems like everything they do aggravates me."

Those who are hurting want to hold someone accountable for the torment they are suffering. Not knowing who to blame, they lash out and become angry at the very ones who want to help. Surprisingly, some authors theorize that anger expressed at the deceased might be essential in helping the mourner to progress toward acceptance of the death (Vargas, Loya, & Hodde-Vargas, 1989). If the anger remains generalized, the griever may not be ready to accept the death and may stagnate, not progressing through the grieving process.

Depression

Depression is expressed as intense sadness and is a normal emotion involved in grief. Even though some degree of depression is experienced by almost all mourners, most do not develop a major depressive episode during the grief experience (Kavanaugh, 1990). Differentiation between depression associated with grief and a major depression is not always easy. According to the American Psychiatric Association's *Diagnostic and Statistical Manual of Mental Disorders* (1994), in comparison to normal bereavement, the person suffering a major depressive disorder will experience one or more of the following symptoms:

- guilt not based on events of the death
- suicidal ideation
- preoccupation with feelings of worthlessness
- hallucinatory experiences other than brief experiences of seeing or hearing the deceased loved one
- obvious impairment in daily functioning
- extreme psychomotor retardation

According to Lightner and Hathaway (1990), those who are experiencing major depression focus on themselves. They see themselves as inadequate and unworthy. Those depressed after the death of a loved one focus on the deceased. They long for the deceased, weep for the deceased, cling to every thought of the deceased. Every act that they perform, every item in their surroundings reminds them of the deceased. Every thought is on the lost love. Everything they do is a painful reminder of their loss (Lightner & Hathaway, 1990). Recurrent episodes of sadness are common for a year or more after bereavement (Parkes & Brown, 1972).

Some who are grieving may withdraw from family and friends. They may become noncommunicative and maintain only minimal association with others. These individuals need solace and privacy as they turn inward to restore harmony and balance to their lives. This type of inward reflection is a positive response for many and is usually short lived.

Guilt

Guilt takes many forms and is often a significant aspect of grief. Those who are hurting want to blame someone or something for the pain and suffering they are experiencing. Because there is really no one to blame, they sometimes blame themselves. This blaming leads to the "If only" syndrome. If only I had . . .

> not let John drive the car . . .

> not given her permission to go . . .

> not said that . . .

> been more cautious, observant, firm,
> compassionate, and so on . . .

then maybe this terrible tragedy could have been prevented. The "If only" syndrome must be faced squarely, examined, and relinquished.

Feelings that generate guilt are many and varied. Guilt is felt because the griever is still alive and can go on with life. Guilt is experienced when the survivor feels he should have done more for the loved one or because relief is felt that the ordeal is over. The survivor must admit these feelings of guilt and forgive himself in order to heal.

Idealization

During the bereavement process, the survivor spends much time reminiscing, reliving past experiences, sharing memories, and thinking about the deceased. In an attempt to avoid painful memories, every recollection portrays the deceased only in the most positive light. The inclination to idealize is so intense that the deceased may appear flawless to the griever. Every negative thought or emotion is suppressed. This experience is called idealization and is a normal part of grieving (Raphael, 1983). Initially, the bereaved is overwhelmed with love and misses the special person enormously. It seems impossible to accept any flaws in the beloved person. However, as time goes by, memories become less selective and a more realistic view surfaces. Acknowledging both the positive and negative qualities of the deceased allows memories to be placed in proper perspective. When the griever assimilates an accurate perception of the deceased, then she is making progress toward successful resolution of grief. If the memory remains distorted or the mourner becomes totally preoccupied with idealization, then the resolution of grief is delayed. With continuance of idealization, relationships with others become difficult and the mourner will live in the past rather than look to the future (Raphael, 1983).

For most people, the process of idealization is positive. It provides the opportunity to review and balance experiences with the loved one. Thoughts and feelings are placed in perspective (Raphael, 1983). Meaning is given to each memory, which helps to restore harmony and peace.

Loneliness

The loss of a spouse causes an inner emptiness or void that leaves the bereaved vulnerable to loneliness. Initially, the survivor may have dinner invitations, be included in social outings, and receive frequent visits. However, as time goes on, the stark reality that this is a couple's world becomes apparent. The visits and the invitations gradually diminish, leaving long days and even longer nights of loneliness. One widow expresses this loneliness in the following vignette.

A Widow's Loneliness

My days are filled with ordinary tasks, cleaning, washing, and so on. I spend much of my day doing the mundane activities that I have always done. However, when I set one place at the dinner table or have no one to discuss the weather or the news with, my heart almost aches with emptiness. But the nights and the evenings are the worst. That's the time when Harry was always home. Our evenings were not glamorous, but quiet. We might work in the yard together, watch a movie, or read. Having no one to share a thought or a laugh with brings the deepest sense of loneliness. Even going to church and sitting alone is painful. I desperately miss the presence of some-one else in the house. I miss being number one in someone's life. I feel so alone.

Great loneliness is also experienced at the death of a child. The parents' world is shattered, empty, and void of meaning. The house is painfully quiet and everything reminds them of their loss. This inner void leaves parents especially vulnerable to the pain of loneliness.

Emotions and the Circle of Human Potentials

Humans were created emotional beings. Emotions should not be despised, ignored, or suppressed. To do this distorts the poten-tial for growth that lies within us all. Keegan and Dossey (1987) developed the Circle of Human Potentials which encompasses five areas: spiritual, mental, emotional, physical, and relationship (see figure 4.1).

Mental, emotional, physical, and relationship potentials con-stantly interact to create a balance in our lives. If any segment becomes distorted, then life is no longer harmonious. With grief, life loses its meaning and this delicate balance is lost. Table 4.2 depicts emotions in each of the areas of human potential that

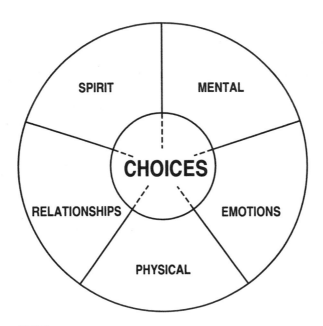

FIGURE 4.1   The circle of human potentials.

Reprinted from Keegan, L., & Dossey, B. 1987. *Self-care: A program to improve your life.* Used with permission of Bodymind Systems, Temple, TX.

Human Potential	Manifestations of Grief
Relationship	Social withdrawal, oversensitivity to behavior of others, difficulty expressing feelings to others
Emotional	Sadness, anger, guilt, anxiety, loneliness, helplessness
Physical	Fatigue, tightness in chest or throat, breathlessness, sleep disturbances, numbness, palpitations, nausea/diarrhea, constipation
Spiritual	Sense of presence of deceased, hallucinations, dreams of the deceased, decrease in ability to pray
Mental	Numbness, disbelief, confusion, inability to make decisions, preoccupation

TABLE 4.2   *Emotional Manifestations of Grief*

play a role in the grieving process. Ideally during the grieving process each emotion that contributes to disharmony is examined and redirected in a more positive form.

The inner circle (see figure 4.1) represents choice. Utilization of the ability to make choices assists one in reaching his fullest potential. In grief, the choice lies not in which emotions are felt, but rather how these emotions are expressed. During the grief experience, emotions must be expressed fully and examined as a search for meaning to the loss is sought. Expression of emotions precedes healing. Healing begins within and moves outward as choices are made that begin to restore equilibrium in all areas of life. In order to heal fully, the self must be nurtured, new relationships must be established, the lost love must be surrendered, and movement must be made toward higher potential. This will restore equilibrium to life.

PROGRESS THROUGH GRIEF

With any death, shock, numbness, and disbelief surface initially. Expressions of shock and numbness include:

"I feel so empty."

"I feel like a robot."

"Time is at a standstill."

"I feel so numb."

"I can't feel anything."

Expressions of disbelief include:

"I must be having a bad dream."

"This can't happen to me."

"This must be a joke!"

"I don't believe it."

These expressions protect the survivor until she is able to face the loss. This phase usually ends with the funeral or shortly thereafter. Until the survivor is able to face the loss, behavior can be mechanical, almost robot-like. Eventually, the reality of the death emerges and the loss must be faced. The following vignette is an account of a young wife's feelings as she emerges from the shock and numbness of the loss of her husband Assam.

Feeling the Loss of Assam

The officer came to the door and told me Assam was not coming home and would never come home. He was dead. An automobile accident had killed him instantly. I felt as if I were dreaming. I heard the baby crying in the back room. Without saying a word to the officer, I closed the door and went to pick up the baby. No tears, no hysteria, no emotion. I held little Sirah in my arms and rocked her until I heard a pounding at the back door. That's how I was the entire week. I was in a trance. I carried on, took care of Sirah, planned the funeral, made the calls, but no emotion.

About a month later, it was as if I suddenly awakened from a deep sleep. It was early in the morning and as I reached across the bed, I realized I was alone. Then overwhelming feelings of desolation and sadness overcame me. I must have sobbed for over an hour. I felt devastated, as if a ton of bricks were on top of me and any minute I would be buried.

Many people mistakenly think that the initial phase of shock and numbness constitutes the entire grieving process. However, as the reality of the death comes into focus, shock and disbelief give way to growing awareness. With awareness, the real pain of grieving begins.

Prevailing thoughts are expressed as follows:

"I felt as though I died as well."

"I felt crushed and devastated."

"I felt abandoned."

"The pain was so deep, so severe."

"My heart was breaking."

Physical symptoms may appear, such as headaches, stomach cramping, chest pain, or difficulty in breathing. Loneliness, guilt, depression, and anger surface. Emotional pain is intense and many times there is the strong desire to tell and retell the details of the death. The griever must be allowed to mourn fully. Emotions must be freely accepted and expressed. Expression provides the opportunity to gain perspective of the loss. Suppression of emotions will prolong grief. With time, recovery occurs as the survivor adapts to living without the loved one. Emotional energy is redirected away from the deceased and reinvested in life. Table 4.3 identifies seven behaviors of the mourner that are indicative of healing. The signs may be subtle at first, but with time full healing occurs.

Shadow Grief

Authors have identified a part of grief called shadow grief (Raphael, 1983). Shadow grief is that intense sadness that overcomes the bereaved when least expected, like a shadow from the past that darkens the day, the moment, or the mood. This reliving of grief may occur at any time, usually at the most unexpected moments, and comes and goes for a lifetime. While

---

The Griever...

Begins to smile spontaneously again

Participates in social activities

Momentarily forgets the death

Begins to view life as pleasurable again

Renews or develops attachments with others

Accepts the death as part of the past

Talks about the deceased with no idealization

▄▄▄

TABLE 4.3 **Seven Signs of Healing**

shadow grief is most often associated with mothers whose children have died, anyone can experience this type of grief (Peppers & Knapp, 1980). A young mother expresses her experience with shadow grief after the death of her daughter, Susan.

Susan's Shadow

Susan died over 2 years ago and for the most part, I am over my grief. I have begun to live again and can see a future without her. Even though my grief has run its course, there are times when this terrible sadness comes over me. It usually happens at the most unexpected times. For instance, last week I was eating lunch at a restaurant, when suddenly I felt totally overcome with grief. Tears flowed down my cheeks and I began to cry. This happens every now and then. I am never prepared for the feeling nor its intensity. I am convinced that Susan's shadow will never leave me. It will always be hidden, waiting to reappear at a moment's notice. In that sense her loss is with me always.

SUMMARY

Surviving the loss of a loved one can be one of life's most difficult challenges. When death severs the relationship with a loved one, the grieving process ensues. The grief that follows the loss of a loved one is a natural response and must be expressed. Grief that is not expressed leads to a disharmony mentally, physically, and spiritually. There are no time frames for grief. While certain aspects of grief are predictable, each individual's journey through the recovery process is unique. Emotional responses surface that are common to all people, without regard to age, sex, or social status. The degree to which these emotional responses are experienced varies greatly from person to person. The nurse-healer can provide families with a knowledge of the normal grief response. This knowledge will assist the griever in understanding what is happening both emotionally and physically. Greater understanding allows the griever to move through the grief to full recovery.

REFLECTIONS

1. Think about the most meaningful relationships in your life.

2. Contemplate the significance of the loss of each of these relationships.

3. Would this loss change your lifestyle? Your circle of friends? Your outlook on life?

4. Would the loss of a loved one cause conflictual relationships to surface?

References

American Psychiatric Association (1994). *Diagnostic and statistical manual of mental disorders* (4th ed.). Washington, DC: Author.

Bugen, L. A. (1977). Human grief: A model for prediction and intervention. *American Journal of Orthopsychiatry, 47,* 196–206.

Hutti, M. (1988, November–December). Perinatal loss: Assisting parents to cope. *Journal of Emergency Nursing, 14(6),* 338–341.

Kavanaugh, D. J. (1990). Towards a cognitive-behavioral intervention for adult grief reactions. *British Journal of Psychiatry, 157,* 373–383.

Keegan, L., & Dossey, B. (1987). *Self-care: A program to improve your life.* Temple, TX: Bodymind Systems.

Kellner, K. R., Donnelly, W. H., & Gould, S. D. (1984). Parental behavior after perinatal death: Lack of predictive demographic and obstetric variables. *Obstetric Gynecology, 63,* 809.

Klass, D. (1986–87). Marriage and divorce among bereaved parents in a self-help group. *Omega, 17,* 237–249.

Lightner, C., & Hathaway, N. (1990). *Giving sorrow words.* New York: Warner Books, Inc.

Parkes, C., & Brown, R. (1972). Health after bereavement: A controlled study of young Boston widows and widowers. *Psychosomatic Medicine, 34,* 449–461.

Peppers, L., & Knapp, R. (1980). Maternal reactions to involuntary fetal/infant death. *Psychiatry, 43,* 155–159.

Powell, J. (1969). *Why am I afraid to tell you who I am?* Niles, IL: Argus Communication.

Raphael, B. (1983). *The anatomy of an illness.* New York: Basic Books, Inc.

Scharlach, A. (1991, April). Factors associated with filial grief following death of an elderly parent. *American Journal of Orthopsychiatry, 61*(2), 307–312.

Schwab, R. (1992). Effects of a child's death on the marital relationship: A preliminary study. *Death Studies, 16,* 141–154.

Vargas, L., Loya, F., & Hodde-Vargas, J. (1989, November). Exploring the multidimensional aspects of grief reactions. *American Journal of Psychiatry, 146*(11), 1484–1488.

5 HELPING CHILDREN COPE WITH GRIEF

Beatriz C. Nieto

Who telleth a tale of unspeaking death?
Who lifteth the veil of what is to come?
Who painteth the shadows that are beneath?
The wide-winding caves of the peopled tomb?
Or uniteth the hopes of what shall be
With the fears and the love for that which we see?

Percy Bysshe Shelley (1792–1822) from "On Death"

Michael and His Grandmother

Ever since he could remember, Michael's grandmother had always been a major part of his life. When he was a baby, she was the one who took care of him while his mom and dad went to work. As he grew a little older, he remembered going on some trips together. They would go to the zoo, to the park, or sometimes they would spend the whole day at the beach. When he started going to school, it was his grandma who would pick him up after school. She would take him home with her until his mom got home from work. Michael enjoyed being with his grandma. They always had lots of fun together. Throughout the years, they had developed a very special bond. Unfortunately, the special relationship that Michael and his grandma enjoyed was cut short because when Michael was nine years old, his grandma died of cancer.

Michael had never really talked to his mom about losing someone special until his grandma became fairly ill. It was during this time that he started to really think about death and that losing his grandma could become a reality. His mom always told him that he shouldn't be afraid to ask about anything that concerned him, and his grandma's health became a major concern for Michael. When he realized that his grandma's health was getting worse, he began asking questions about her health. He wanted to know if his grandma was ever going to get better or was she going to die and if she were, when was it going to happen? Michael also asked his mom why his grandma had to die. Deep down inside he did not want her to die and just thinking about losing his grandma made him feel very sad. Although his mom tried to answer his questions as thoroughly and honestly as she could, he continued to ask the same questions. He hoped that his mom would tell him that his grandma was going to get better and that she was not going to die. Unfortunately, that was not so. His grandma died two years after being diagnosed with cancer.

After his grandma's death, Michael continued to be full of questions, such as, "Now that grandma is gone, what will happen to her body?" "Will I ever see her again?" "Can grandma still see me?" "Where is heaven?" "Am I going to die?" and "Mom, are you going to die too?"

INTRODUCTION

If you have ever been around a child or have one or more of your own, you know that they are constantly asking questions. Who? What? Where? When? and Why? are just a few that come up during a normal interaction with a child. It seems they have a never-ending supply of questions. Normally we try to answer their questions as best we can, hoping that our answers will be sufficient to satisfy their curiosity. Often, depending on the age of the child, we are lucky enough to get away with answering their questions without having to come up with long, elaborate explanations. Other times, however, a child's question may require more detail than we may be ready or willing to give.

Have you ever been confronted by a child asking questions about death and dying? Have you ever wondered if you could handle answering such questions? Some of us may feel that it is hard enough to answer ordinary questions without having to worry about answering questions concerning death and dying. Eventually, we may all face the task of answering questions asked by a child about death and dying. Once a child begins asking questions about death and dying, there is no way to avoid the situation. They need answers to their questions and so do we. When we come face to face with a situation dealing with death and dying, we may have questions of our own— questions that need answering. For example, "How should we answer their questions?" "How much detail should we tell them?" "How can I best help my child through this situation?" "Is there anyone who can help me?" These were some questions that Michael's mom faced when his grandma died of cancer. Not only did she have to deal with her grief over the loss of her mother, but she had to be sensitive to the needs of Michael. This was a difficult task since Michael had never experienced the loss of someone so close to his heart. Though Michael's mom had been a nurse for many years and had her share of dealing with death and dying, she did not feel fully prepared for the loss of her mother and the task of helping Michael to cope with his grief. She relied on what she had learned in nursing school and from life itself, but never had she felt so vulnerable and so inadequate and at times so desperate. This was especially true when she would find Michael crying quietly in his room, missing his grandma so much.

This chapter focuses on children and how they deal with death and dying. How they cope with the loss of a loved one and how we as adults can help them through their grief are also explored. This is done by presenting viewpoints on how children learn and how, through experiences that occur throughout their life cycle, they develop and learn about death and dying. Also presented are some psychological tasks a child may experience as he progresses through the grieving process. The last part of this chapter focuses on helping the child cope with the loss.

CHILDREN AND DEATH

The topic of death and dying is never an easy subject for discussion. Often, just the thought of someone we love dying can make us feel uncomfortable and cause feelings of sadness. Because it is one of the most difficult topics to think about, there may be a tendency to repress and turn away from it until we are in a situation that forces us to come face to face with an actual death.

When death occurs in a family, it affects every member of that family in one way or another. The children, depending on their ages and relationship to the deceased, are also affected by the death. How do we deal with children when a death in the family has occurred? Often the initial reaction of the adults is to protect the children by not exposing them to the different aspects of the situation caused by the death. We as adults need to be comfortable with our own feelings of death and dying, our faith, and our own mortality. Becoming comfortable with our own feelings is important before attempting to understand what children know, how they learn about death and dying, and how we can help them cope with the situation.

Throughout history, attempts to understand how children learn have been introduced. Plato, in the fourth century B.C., believed that all knowledge exists within a person from birth. John Locke, a seventeenth-century English philosopher, argued that a child knows absolutely nothing before birth and that learning occurs through experience. Although these philosophers varied in their ideas of learning, today psychological evidence suggests that the theories of both these philosophers are important components of learning. Lifton and Olson (1974) stated that modern psychological evidence suggests that a "child does have a kind of knowledge at birth, and that this 'knowledge' is vastly extended and made concrete only by experience with the environment" (p. 42). They believed that this concept of death gradually emerges from the "inner imagery that the child apparently has at birth and is developed and made concrete in relation to the child's experiences" (p. 46). They also said that the child's imagery and ideas associated with death continue to evolve over the course of the life cycle and these ideas reflect both the child's individual experiences and the development of intellectual capacities.

To help us better understand the child's earliest imagery of life and death, Lifton and Olson (1974) explained the imagery of death and dying by using three sets of opposite concepts. They are as follows:

1. connection—separation

2. movement—stasis (lack of movement)

3. integrity—disintegration (p. 46)

Connection—Separation

When a child is born, there is a natural bonding that occurs between the infant and her mother. As the infant matures and develops, she soon realizes that one person is her mother and when she is with this person, she is most content. The connection component of the first pair of opposites is created because of the infant's dependence on her mother to help meet all her needs. The imagery surrounding the relationship between the child and her mother is developed because of the child's expectation for nourishment and care from the mother. This expectation for nourishment and care stimulates further seeking of attachment by the child to her mother. Therefore, it can be concluded that the infant's life is dependent on being *connected* to the source of care and support.

On the other hand, the counterpart to the connection component is *separation*. Separation of the child from his parents may result in producing feelings of extreme fear and anxiety in the child. The image that occurs when the child is left alone or separated from the source of his nurturing can be described as an initial association to an image of death and loss. This may be the beginning of the child experiencing and learning about death and dying.

Movement—Stasis (Lack of Movement)

Play and exercise are important parts of a child's everyday existence. By engaging in various kinds of play and exercise, the child can grow and develop not only her mind, but her physical body as well. As the child's muscles develop, so does her muscle coordination, which in turn increases her ability to move about more freely. The concept of *movement* in this set of opposites is seen as representing motion, energy, and life itself.

The other component in this set of opposites is defined by *stasis*, or lack of movement. It is this concept that Lifton and Olson (1974) believed the child associates with the imagery of death. Since movement is associated with life, a child who is held still against his will may respond by becoming overwrought and distressed at not being able to move freely. The child, therefore, may equate this inability to move with death. Since a child may equate the inability to move with death and because during sleep he is least in motion, equating death with sleep in not uncommon in a child. Further encouragement of this association between sleep and death may come from other sources such as nighttime prayers. For example, this is evident in one well-known nighttime prayer that begins as follows:

> Now I lay me down to sleep,
> I pray the Lord my soul to keep.
> If I should die before I wake,
> I pray the Lord my soul to take.

As parents, we might not want our children to be exposed to such prayers because of the context and because this is not considered the best way to teach children about death. Lifton and Olson (1974) pointed out, however, that in some situations, the association of sleep with death can make death less frightening for a child. An example of this can be seen in the following vignette:

Annie

Annie, a 3 1/2 year old, stayed with her grandmother while her mother worked. One day, as usual, Annie's mother came to pick her up from her grandmother's house. She found Annie in the bedroom laying by her grandmother, who had suffered a fatal heart attack just a few hours earlier. Annie's mother was shocked and at first thought that something had happened to both of them. As she got closer to where they both laid, Annie quietly opened her eyes. She whispered softly that her grandma had gone to sleep on the floor and that she had gone to sleep as well.

This vignette depicts a very young child equating death with sleep. Because this child equated death with sleep, it seemed not to bother her that her grandmother was not moving, and in fact had died. It is only with time that a child will become able to distinguish the difference between death and sleep and realize the finality of death. For example, the preschool child may think of death as reversible. She may think that the person who died has gone away but will return. A much older child begins to realize that not only is death final, but inevitable and that no one, including himself, is immune from it.

It is important to remember that the age in which the child will begin to understand the imagery of death and dying will vary with each individual child. Lifton and Olson (1974) stated that usually, the ages in which understanding of death occurs are between 5 and 9, but further emphasized that "children begin to become aware of death much earlier than this, although their ideas may be vague and confused" (p. 48).

Integrity—Disintegration

In this set of opposites, *integrity* of life is described as staying in one piece or keeping oneself intact. *Disintegration*, on the other hand, means falling apart or going to pieces. From very early in life, the focus of integrity and/or disintegration is on one's body or self-image. Children tend to have strong feelings of fear that bodily annihilation and disintegration will occur. These reactions are evident when a child experiences a cut, injury, or sees blood. A child's reaction may seem exaggerated, but to him, a simple cut or scrape, especially when bleeding is a factor, may be associated with the fear of disintegration or falling apart. He may think he is going to bleed to death, or that all his insides will ooze out through the cut or scrape.

Lifton and Olson (1974) stated that the fears of disintegration and bodily annihilation "are related to fears of separation and stasis, since all death imagery is bound closely together" (p. 48). They further stated that "situations that relate to imagery of separation, stasis, and disintegration cause extreme anxiety even when the experiences themselves are not actually dangerous" and to understand these exaggerated fears, we need to see them in the more ultimate image of extinction to which they relate (p. 49). That is to say that there is a life-death imagery that endures and evolves throughout life. At the moment of birth, a child's innate potential for death imagery is begun, since she is no longer in her mother's safe and secure womb. The infant finds herself suddenly taken away from her mother, vulnerable to pain and to the fear of disintegration. As the infant grows and develops through each stage of the life cycle, she will again experience the vulnerability and fears of disintegration. This is thought to occur because the beginning of each new stage of development signifies a new beginning. An individual will again be faced with certain anxieties and uncertainties. Lifton and Olson (1974) pointed out that "each new step or each new 'birth' on the way to becoming a fully developed person will rekindle the death anxieties associated with the innate imagery of separation, stasis, and disintegration" (p. 49).

GRIEF PROCESS IN CHILDREN

Baker, Sedney, and Gross (1992) conceptualized the grief process in children as a series of tasks that must be accomplished over a period of time. These tasks are categorized into three major phases. The first category of tasks is referred to as the early tasks, which begin when the child first learns of the death. During these early tasks, the child's major goals are to gain understanding of what has occurred and incorporate self-protective mechanisms. This will help shield him from the full emotional impact of the loss. The second category of tasks is referred to as the middle-phase tasks. It is during this time that the child's goals include "accepting and reworking the loss and bearing the intense psychological pain involved" (Baker et al., 1992, p. 105). The third category of tasks is referred to as the late tasks. These tasks occur when the child focuses on reclaiming sense of who she is and resuming her developmental progress.

In order for the child to progress through these tasks sequentially, the earlier tasks must be accomplished in a satisfactory manner before the later tasks can be addressed. Therefore, as Baker et al. (1992) pointed out, "the grief process will not progress until the tasks of each stage are addressed and accomplished" (p. 106).

Early Tasks

In order for a child to begin to grieve, he must know that a death has occurred. He must feel assured that his own safety is not at risk. Baker et al. (1992) pointed out that "the early tasks of grieving are focused on (1) understanding the fact that someone has died and the implications of this fact and (2) self-protection of themselves, their bodies, and their families" (p. 106). It is important to point out at this time that in order for a child to have any chance of mastering the experience of the loss, the child must be equipped with general knowledge of death and dying and about the particular situation in which the death has occurred. Children normally get their information by listening intently, watching the reactions of others, and asking questions. If a child's questions are not answered accurately or thoroughly, as necessary for the child's age, the child may be inclined to fill the missing pieces with her imagination. It is important to remember that even when giving a child the information she requires, an adequate amount of time should be allowed for the child to process the information gradually. The child should be provided with accurate information in age-appropriate language to help her grasp both the intellectual and emotional meaning of the loss.

The second portion of the early tasks deals with that of personal safety issues for the child. Furman (1974) stated that not only is it necessary for the child to understand death, but he needs to feel safe in a secure environment. Oftentimes, when a death has occurred, children may fear that they, too, will die, and that their family will no longer exist. When the child or his family as a whole feels unable to survive, the difficult task of grieving cannot begin. Self-protective mechanisms may come into play at this time. The child and/or his family may use denial, distortion, and emotional or physical isolation from others as self-protective mechanisms. All his energy goes into protecting the other members of the family.

Middle-Phase Tasks

Baker et al. (1992) characterized the middle phase of grief with the following three tasks:

- accepting and emotionally acknowledging the reality of the loss
- exploring and reevaluating the relationship to the lost love object
- facing and bearing the psychological pain that accompanies the realization of the loss (p. 109)

This phase of grief includes the mourning process in which all aspects of the relationship to the deceased will be explored in great detail. Aspects of the relationship explored by the individual who has suffered a loss will include those of gratification, ambivalence, and disappointments. This is true for both adults and children. It is during this phase that painful feelings of loss and despair set in because of having accepted the idea that the person is truly gone. The child must endure this despair to successfully complete this phase of tasks and continue satisfactorily with the grief process.

Late Tasks

As was stated earlier, the tasks in the third phase of grieving are related to the reorganization of the child's sense of identity and of significant relationships in her life. In further delineating the tasks included in this phase of the grief process, Baker et al. (1992) listed five steps a child must go through to help accomplish the tasks involved in the late phase of the grief process. They are as follows:

- The child must evolve a new sense of personal identity that includes the experience of the loss and some identifications with the deceased.

- The child needs to invest in new emotional relationships without an excessive fear of loss and without a constant need to compare the new person to the dead person.

- The child must be able to consolidate and maintain a durable internal relationship of the lost love object that will survive over time in such a way that the lost love object becomes a new type of sustaining inner presence for the child.

- The child must be able to return wholeheartedly to age-appropriate developmental tasks and activities, thus resuming the developmental course that was interrupted by the emotional loss.

- The child must be able to cope with the periodic resurgence of painful affect, usually at points of developmental transition or on specific anniversaries, such as the date of the person's death. (p. 111)

The conceptualization of the grief process, as presented by Baker et al. (1992), described the course of a child's grief reaction over time. It is imperative, however, that we understand that it does not mean that these reactions will emerge in a simple linear manner from the early tasks to the later ones (p. 115). From time to time, the child may experience certain relapses. It is during these regressions that "the child may return to tasks that were addressed earlier, but were not completely resolved" (p. 115). The occurrence of these regressions is seen more frequently around the time of developmental transitions of the child.

HELP FOR THE GRIEVING CHILD

As was stated earlier, the subject of death and dying is never easy to talk about. This is especially true when it means thinking about losing someone you love. People are not comfortable with the subject and do not like talking about death. This was not the case in the past. Because we were once more of an agrarian society than we are today, children were exposed to the realities of the natural life cycle of plants and animals. People often died in the home, and family members grieved together. Death was seen as being a part of life. Nowadays, this is seldom the case. It is unfortunate that "death is a subject that is evaded, ignored, and denied by our youth worshiping, progress-oriented society" (Kübler-Ross, 1975, p. 10).

It is this mentality that we need to overcome in order for us to come to grips with the realities of death and be instrumental in helping our children learn and cope with the loss of someone they love. In order for us, as adults, to understand and help our children cope with death, there are certain facts pertaining to young grievers that need to be taken into consideration. The facts characterizing young grievers are outlined in table 5.1.

These facts have been developed and used primarily with children who have experienced the death of a parent, but they can also be applied to a variety of situations in which a child has suffered a loss. Being aware of these facts can help us to become better prepared when faced with a situation involving a child who has suffered a loss and is experiencing grief. For it is in us that our children seek the answers to their questions. Our feelings and attitude toward death and loss are quickly sensed and assimilated by our children. We need to maintain a pattern of honesty and openness to help ease the pain and strengthen the bonds with others.

It is believed that the timing of children's grief reactions will often follow closely on the timing of their parents' grieving (Baker et al., 1992). Furman (1974) pointed out that the grief process in children is heavily dependent on parental support. It is imperative that this adult parental support be constant, for any interruption may cause the grief process to be suspended during the time that support is not available. This may prevent the child from progressing into the later tasks of the grief process.

One of the most important ways to help our children through the grief process is through communication. How and what we communicate with our children is of vital importance. We have to get over our reluctance to talk to our children about

- Young people ask three questions about the death of a parent:
  Did I cause the death in any way? (Being disobedient, etc.)
  Who will take care of me?
  Will death ever happen to me?

- Young people have a delayed reaction to grief.

- Different relationships to the deceased parent have an impact on grieving. An ambivalent relationship may cause guilt. Young people also "grieve for what might have been."

- Many young people are concerned if they are grieving right and tend to repress their grief. Having limited experiences with death they do not know what to expect.

- Other young people may be too scared to reach out to a friend who has lost a parent because they think it may happen to them. The young griever may need the support of a peer group that have shared similar death experiences.

- Young people cannot verbalize their feeling and often times cover up their real feelings. Young grievers, especially boys, give mixed messages about their grief to retain a "macho" image. Actions rather than words are more appropriate for a young person.

- A young person may be concerned about demonstrating sadness as not to upset other family members. Silence and withdrawal can be interpreted as not caring.

- Developmental maturity has a great deal to do with grieving. Many aspects of grief are misunderstood because of the lack of maturity. As the child matures to another developmental stage, the death is reprocessed. New questions will arise at each new stage.

- Young people often do not have the close friends or support systems that can assist them in learning about the grieving process. It is important for them to come to a support group to learn about grief and to realize their feelings are normal.

TABLE 5.1   *Facts to Be Considered Concerning Young Grievers*

Used with permission from Louise M. Aldrich, MSW, Children's Bereavement Counselor, Samaritan Hospice, Moorestown, NJ.

death. We need to realize that our children may understand more about death than we think they do. It is important to remember that a child's concept of death will vary depending on his age and developmental stage. For example, an infant's and toddler's greatest fears focus on becoming separated from their parents. Even though they may not be old enough to have a concrete understanding of the concept of death, playing a simple game like peek-a-boo with a child may be the beginning of the development of the death imagery that Lifton and Olson (1974) spoke about. Preschoolers, whose ages may range from 3 to 5 years, may associate death with sleep and think of it as being temporary and reversible. Since their way of thinking involves fantasy and imagination, preschoolers may think that the dead person has gone away but will return. They may also think that the person will once again get up and walk, even though she is dead. It is between the ages of 5 and 9 that children begin to gradually realize that death is irreversible, ubiquitous, and private. By age 9 or 10 a child understands the finality of death, that it is inevitable, and that everyone, including them, will someday die.

Helping a child understand death is a lifelong process and not an easy task to accomplish. Our abilities to be open and honest about death may be hindered because we may have been brought up in households that did not talk openly about death. Our parents may have thought it best if we were not exposed to the realities of death. This may have been their way of protecting us, or it may have been their way of protecting themselves from having to face questions they were not prepared to answer. So how can we as parents prepare ourselves?

Preparation is a key element in learning to help our children learn and understand death. Helping children deal with death early in life will help them grow and develop good coping skills. These coping skills will become the essence of being able to cope with death throughout their lifetime. Table 5.2 illustrates some do's and don'ts developed by Kuenning (1987) that focus on what we as adults can do to help our children understand death. Her ideas focus on helping children understand death by exposing them to different concepts that may occur before, during, and after a death. These ideas can be utilized by everyone and can be applied to different situations. They illustrate practical ways in which we can help our children understand death.

There are also other ways we can use to help a child through the grieving process. Some of the ways in which we can help children not only express their feelings but also help themselves heal is by encouraging them to participate in writing and art activities (Aldrich, 1993). Some of the suggested ways may include keeping a journal, writing poems, stories, or biographies, or making a collage of magazine pictures or words that remind

---

DO'S

1. Teach with animals and plants. When a pet dies, a child mourns. By doing so, the child is developing the ability to work through grief. This experience will give your child the opportunity to gain a gradual understanding of human death. Don't replace the animal right away.

   You can also use the life cycle of plants to teach about death. The same language is used for plants (plants live, plants grow, plants die) as for all living things.

2. Be open to a child's questioning about death. Don't avoid or change the subject. Children need to know it is not a closed subject. If you don't know the answer, say, "I don't know." Talk about death without fear or denial. The unknown is what children fear most, for it stirs anxiety and fantasy. It is wise to talk naturally about death with a child before it impacts them personally. Read books about death with them. Arm your child with knowledge before he or she is faced with a crisis.

3. Give accurate information promptly and be honest. There is usually a precise reason for death. Children will want to know everything and therefore, we need to remain open and honest throughout the situation.

4. Ask what truth the child is seeking. We may assume they want a lot of information when a simple fact will do. Don't assume; answer questions with questions until you are able to find out what it is they are really asking. Begin with where the child is and only answer what they ask.

5. Use "death" language; avoid euphemisms. Say, "he died," rather than "he passed away" or "we lost him." Euphemisms are vague and create confusion in understanding. By misunderstanding common adult expressions, children frequently arrive at serious misconceptions.

6. Differentiate between minor illness and fatal illness. Children learn that other children die, but you need to reassure them that it is only when a child is very sick or has an accident they die. Most children grow up and live to be old.

7. Do expose the child to the dying person. With guidance and support from parents, sometimes it is helpful for a youngster to share in the process of watching a person die. The dying person can minister to loved ones, as is often done in the hospice setting.

8. Explain the terminal illness. Explain to them the treatment regimen and let them know that everything possible is being done to help their loved one.

9. Reassure the child that he or she will be cared for and not abandoned if the dying person is a parent. If you are the surviving parent, reassure your child that you are taking care of yourself and probably won't die until you are old. It is important, however, that children know that everybody will die someday. It is vitally important for parents to have a will and guardianship assigned for their children in the event of simultaneous death of both parents. It is wise to discuss this with your children.

10. Give the child the option of attending the funeral and other religious rituals. Never force, but do encourage. When parents deny them participation in funeral procedures, the children feel isolated and burdened by confusion and by unexpressed grief. By viewing the body and seeing the casket left at the cemetery answers some questions the child has about where the body has gone.

TABLE 5.2   *How to Help Your Child Understand Death*

11. Be aware of irrational guilt feelings. Reassure the child that he or she did not cause the death and could not have stopped its happening. Children need to be told that their bad thoughts toward a loved one did not cause death.

12. Give the child affection. Be nonverbal and open to physically comforting your child.

13. Be open about your tears and feelings. Say, "I feel very sad because Grandpa died." Let the child know that you will not always feel this way. Don't pretend as though nothing has happened.

14. Encourage reminiscing about the deceased. Remembering good times and wonderful things about the person who has died creates memories that help the child accept the death.

15. Encourage the child to write a letter or draw pictures. Experts say the very act of writing letters to the survivor, to God, or to the deceased is a way for children to heal emotional hurts.

16. Speak of heaven in terms of relationship with God rather than a place. Tell them, "Heaven is where God is. 'God is love' and the life of heaven is a life of love. Children understand this; they know that nothing is more important than love" (Reed, 1970, p. 30).

17. Pray for wisdom. Ask God to direct you in knowing how to respond to your child's questions about death.

DONT'S

---

1. Avoid judgmental statements and don't moralize. Don't say, "You mustn't say that," or "Don't feel that way." Don't tell the child how he or she should feel.

2. Don't equate death with sleep or sickness. The child may confuse sleep with death because he or she recognizes both states as being still. He needs reassurance that death is not a long sleep. The sleep he takes each night is rest.

3. Don't say, "God needed her," or "God took her," or "God punished her," or that "It is God's will." It is unwise to tell a child that God wanted their loved one. The child may feel that God may want him next. Assure your child God is sorry when tragedies happen and that He understands our pain and will help us through it.

4. Don't fragment the family or initiate more change than necessary. Try to maintain the family routine as much as possible to reinforce feelings of security.

5. Don't use the child as a "parent replacement" for a lost spouse. Nor should the parent assign to the child the absent parent's role. Don't say, "Now you are the 'man' or 'woman' of the house." This is an unfair burden and robs the child of his or her child-hood. It is assigning the child an impossible task.

6. Don't try to stop the grieving process. Be accepting. Give the child permission to grieve. To help prevent future emotional difficulties, encourage the child to talk about feelings of grief such as fear, anger, guilt, and loneliness. Explain that these feelings are appropriate and normal, and so is crying. Allowing the child to grieve, openly and freely, will allow him to move from hurt to health.

TABLE 5.2   *How to Help Your Child Understand Death (continued)*

From *Helping People Through Grief* by Dolores Kuenning, 1987, Minneapolis, MN: Bethany House Publishers. Copyright 1987 by Bethany House Publishers. Reprinted with permission.

the child of the person. These activities can be both beneficial and instrumental in allowing the child to express herself in other ways, besides verbally.

The importance of helping a child through the grieving process cannot be overemphasized. Not only do we need to be aware of our children's feelings and how they are coping with the loss, but we have to be sensitive to the fact that they may not be able to handle the situation. Besides helping the child express his feelings and work through the grieving process, we also need to be aware of abnormal reactions that may occur when a child is not able to progress satisfactorily. Some of the abnormal grief reactions as described by Aldrich (1989) are outlined in table 5.3.

Aldrich (1989) stated that we need to familiarize ourselves with these reactions in order to identify children that may be exhibiting them and may need professional counseling. She

---

- anger toward anyone and everyone

- excessive misbehaving or fighting

- indifference to activities the young person used to enjoy

- constant physical ailments

- running away from home

- truancy

- rejecting family, friends, authority

- having difficulty relaxing

- using drugs or alcohol

- constant anxiety

- constant depression and wanting to be alone

- self-blame or guilt

- inability or unwillingness to talk about the person who died

- talk of reunion with the person who died or a desire to die

---

TABLE 5.3   *Abnormal Grief Reactions in Children*

Used with permission from Louise M. Aldrich, MSW, Children's Bereavement Counselor, Samaritan Hospice, Moorestown, NJ.

emphasizes that these reactions may be cries for help, especially when they become intense, last a long time, or both (p. 42). Fox (1988) stated that "it is often possible to talk with a troubled, bereaved youngster and determine if he or she is stuck on the task of understanding, grieving, commemorating, or going on" (p. 11). She further states that it is important for "children and adolescents to accomplish these four psychological tasks if their grief is to be *good grief*—that is, grief that helps them grow and develop good coping skills" (p. 10).

SUMMARY

One of the biggest challenges that we will be faced with is dealing with the death of someone we know. That, in itself, may prove to be the most difficult and stressful event we will come face to face with throughout our lifetime. In fact, it may be a situation in which our mind, body, and soul will be put through the test of enduring pain, loneliness, and grief as a result of having lost someone close to our heart. We have to search deep within ourselves in order to be able to survive and go on with our lives. This is especially true if children are involved. For it is in us that children seek their answers. Whether we want to be or not, we are their role models. It is our example that they will follow. If we are comfortable with our feelings and are not afraid to show our emotions and our grief, then our children will more than likely do the same. If we are not able to deal with the situation or answer their questions honestly, they may not be able to accomplish the necessary tasks that are a vital part of the grieving process. It is up to us to "identify issues that may be making it difficult for children and adolescents to deal with the death" (Fox, 1988, p. 11). Seeking help from other sources, e.g., schools, camps, religious groups and community organizations that are prepared and trained to assist the grieving child, may become necessary.

It is important to remember that we need to be honest with ourselves as well as our children. We need to become comfortable with our own feelings about all the realities concerning death and dying. Maintaining open lines of communication and answering our children's questions about death and dying as thoroughly and consistently as possible is of vital importance. For

Do I . . .	Yes	No
• remember significant losses as a young person/adult?	____	____
• talk about these significant losses?	____	____
• discuss death comfortably?	____	____
• remember a relative/close friend dying?	____	____
• attend the funerals of people I know who have died?	____	____
• deal well with emotions/feelings of grief?	____	____
• remember my feelings when I learned death was final?	____	____
• recognize my feelings about death now?	____	____

If you have consistent negative answers on this guide, it may indicate that more about death, dying, and grief is needed.

TABLE 5.4   Death Sensitivity Guide

Used with permission from Louise M. Aldrich, MSW, Children's Bereavement Counselor, Samaritan Hospice, Moorestown, NJ.

when we become comfortable with our own mortality, then we can become instrumental in helping our children grow and develop the skills they need to cope with the realities of life.

REFLECTIONS

A prerequisite for any adult intent on helping a bereaved child through the grief process is learning how she as an adult feels about death or loss. As adults, we often feel uncomfortable dealing with death. The Death Sensitivity Guide (table 5.4) may help us realize that before we assist young people, we may need more education and training concerning the grief process.

References

Aldrich, L. M. (1989). *CANS: Children adjusting to new situations. A grief support group program for children who have experienced the death of a parent.* Moorestown, NJ: Samaritan Hospice.

Aldrich, L. M. (1993, February). The grieving child: Helping your students cope with death. *Learning*, 40–43.

Baker, J. E., Sedney, M. A., & Gross, E. (1992). Psychological tasks for bereaved children. *American Journal of Orthopsychiatry, 62*(1), 105–116.

Fox, S. S. (1988, August). Helping the child deal with death teaches valuable skills. *The Psychiatric Times*, 10–12.

Furman, E. (1974). *A child's parent dies: Studies in childhood bereavement.* New Haven, CT: Yale University Press.

Kübler-Ross, E. (1975). *Death: The final stage of growth.* Englewood Cliffs, NJ: Prentice-Hall.

Kuenning, D. (1987). *Helping people through grief.* Minneapolis: Bethany House.

Lifton, R. J., & Olson, E. (1974). *Living and dying.* New York: Praeger Publishers.

Reed, E. L. (1970). *Helping children with the mystery of death.* Nashville: Abingdon Press.

6 | AIDS AND GRIEVING

Beatriz C. Nieto

Do not go gentle into that good night,
Old age should burn and rave at close of day;
Rage, rage against the dying of the light.

Dylan Thomas

Aurelia

Aurelia Martinez has been in a long-term monogamous relationship
with her husband of 9 years, Reynaldo. Recently, Reynaldo has experienced chronic fatigue, and has swollen lymph nodes; his doctor
suggests that he and Aurelia be tested for HIV. Aurelia protests that
they have been faithful to each other, and she reluctantly agrees to
the test. When both test positive, Reynaldo tells her that before he
met her, he had been sexually active with both men and women.
Of their two children, Jaime's test result was positive and Raquel's
was negative.

Stephen

Stephen is holding on to his lover of 5 years, John, who is dying of AIDS. It seems just a few years ago they were making plans for the future. Now it seems that nothing is certain. Stephen finds himself feeling guilty over his partner's illness; angry with his impending death, and fearful of what is to come.

Lucy

Lucy, a nurse on 5-East is expecting another admission, a 35-year-old with the diagnosis of AIDS. The nurse is new to the unit and has never taken care of a patient with AIDS before. She feels overwhelmed and asks herself if she can provide care for this patient.

INTRODUCTION

At times, it is unbelievable to think that over a decade has passed since the human immunodeficiency virus (HIV) infection was first officially and clinically recognized. Even more alarming are the deadly consequences of HIV infection that culminate in the diagnosis of the acquired immunodeficiency syndrome (AIDS). As we embark into the second decade of this dreaded disease, it is overwhelming to consider the deadly consequences and the devastation AIDS has managed to create. What was once a new and unfamiliar phenomenon has become one of the most cataclysmic and rampant health crises to spread to all corners of the world. From its inception, HIV has touched and changed the lives of many. The disease, which was once thought to afflict only young homosexual men, is now affecting people from all walks of life, including an alarming increase in women and children. The following story tells of losing a childhood friend to AIDS.

Oscar's Story

Oscar was our neighbor. We both lived in the same apartment complex. He was 5 years old when we first met him, the same age as my younger sister. Oscar was a hemophiliac and had to have multiple blood transfusions when he was very young. To look at him, no one would have known that he was sick. He was fair skinned and had blond hair. He was a sweet boy, a picture of an angel. At the age of 13, he began to get sick a lot. We noticed that he stopped coming to visit us and that he spent more time at the hospital. In 1988, at the age of 14, Oscar died of AIDS-related complications. I will never forget the shock and anger I felt when we found out about his death. I remember thinking how unfair it was. He was too young and had never really gotten a chance to experience life and do exciting things. It seemed that all his life he was confined to blood transfusion and factor VIII for his hemophilia. He had to be careful in everything he did. Despite what little he could do, I still remember he was a happy child, full of love. In the end he lost his life, not to his hemophilia, but to something that no one knew existed a few years before. He did nothing wrong, yet he suffered most of his young life. I will always remember the fair-skinned, blond kid who loved life in spite of all its unfairness.

AIDS seems to have no boundaries and thus far, no cure. AIDS is known to attack and debilitate young, healthy people and is uniformly fatal. It is a killer of youth and affects the very being of the person who is unfortunate enough to become afflicted with this deadly disease. AIDS forces many to live in dreadful anticipation of a horrible death and leaves many to mourn the death of loved ones. It has forced some parents to face the untimely reality of losing their children. This chapter is written with these thoughts in mind. The chapter's focus is on different aspects of loss and grief as they relate to nursing and the AIDS epidemic.

THE AIDS EPIDEMIC

AIDS has been characterized as the most severe disease state on a continuum of illnesses related to infection by the retrovirus HIV (Flaskerud, 1989). Piemme and Bolle (1990) described AIDS as a "life-threatening condition characterized by a serious impairment of the cell-mediated branch of the immune system, which leaves the person defenseless against infections and certain forms of malignancies" (p. 266). Nuland (1994) stated that "medical science has never before confronted a microbe that destroys the very cells of the immune system whose job it is to coordinate the body's resistance to it; immunity against a swarming score of secondary invaders is defeated before it has had a chance to mount a defense" (p. 172).

The first recognized cases of AIDS occurred in the summer of 1981 when previously healthy people were diagnosed with pneumocystis carinii pneumonia (PCP) and Kaposi's sarcoma (KS). Both conditions had been seen in severely immunocompromised individuals before this time (Curran, Morgan, & Hardy, 1985). It is important to realize that opportunistic infections are a formidable foe for those infected with the AIDS virus. Pathogens that threaten the lives of patients with the HIV infection exist everywhere in nature. It is impossible for these patients to avoid exposure to these pathogens (Ungvarski & Schmidt, 1992).

HIV disease manages to make the human immune system itself the primary target for its attack. The immune response affected is the one dependent on the helper T lymphocytes (T_4/CD_4 cells). It reproduces inside the T_4 cell and destroys them (Burris, Dalton, Miller & the Yale AIDS Law Project, 1993, p. 21). The Centers for Disease Control (1993) have developed a group classification system for HIV infection according to clinical conditions and T_4/CD_4 cell counts. They have also expanded the case definition for advanced HIV disease or AIDS (see table 6.1).

T₄/CD₄ Categories

Category 1: $\geq$ 500 cells/μL	Category 2: 200–499 cells/μL	Category 3: < 200 cells/μL

Clinical Categories

Category A   Categories B and C have not occurred

                  Asymptomatic HIV infection

                  Persistent generalized lymphadenopathy

                  Acute (primary) HIV infection

Category B   Category C has not occurred

                  Conditions attributed to HIV infection indicative of a deficient cell-mediated immune system

                  Conditions considered by physician to have a clinical course or require management that is complicated by HIV infection

        Examples of Category B conditions include but are not limited to the following:

Bacillary angiomatosis	Oral hairy leukoplakia
Candidiasis, oropharyngeal (thrush)	Herpes zoster
Candidiasis, vulvovaginal	Idiopathic thrombocytopenic purpura
Cervial dysplasia	Listeriosis
Constitutional symptoms such as fever	Pelvic inflammatory disease
or diarrhea for more than 1 month	Peripheral neuropathy

Category C   All clinical conditions listed as advanced HIV disease or AIDS (Once in category C, the person remains in this category).

AIDS Case Definition

The AIDS surveillance case has been expanded to include persons with T₄/CD₄ lymphocyte count below 200 cells/μL or T₄/CD₄ percentage below 14 or with previous clinical conditions in the 1987 AIDS case definition, with the inclusion of pulmonary tuberculosis (MTB), recurrent pneumonia, and invasive cervical cancer. The following are the AIDS-defining illnesses according to the CDC guidelines:

Candidiasis of esophagus, trachea, bronchi, and lungs	Lymphoma, immunoblastic
	Lymphoma of brain
Cervical cancer, invasive	Mycobacterium avium-intracellulare or
Coccidioidomycosis, disseminated or extrapulmonary	M. kansasii, disseminated or extrapulmonary
	Mycobacterium tuberculosis, any site
Cryptococcosis outside of lungs	(pulmonary or extrapulmonary)
Cryptosporidial diarrhea for over 1 month	Mycobacterium, other species, disseminated or
Herpes simplex causing skin ulcers for over 1 month, pneumonia, bronchitis, or esophagitis	extrapulmonary
	Pneumocystis carinii pneumonia
	Pneumonia, recurrent
Histoplasmosis, disseminated or extrapulmonary	Progressive multifocal leukoencephalopathy
Isosporiasis, chronic diarrhea for over 1 month	(PML)
Kaposi's sarcoma in patients less than 60 years of age	Salmonella septicemia, recurrent
	Toxoplasmic encephalitis
Lymphoma, Burkitt's	Wasting syndrome caused by HIV

TABLE 6.1   *Classification System for HIV Infection*

Centers for Disease Control (1993). 1993 revised classification system for HIV infection and expanded surveillance case definition for AIDS among adolescents and adults, MMWR 41 (RR-17): 1.

AIDS Transmission

The transmission of HIV infection is the result of exchange of body fluids, especially blood, semen, vaginal fluid, and mothers' milk. Three methods of HIV transmission are (1) intimate sexual contact; (2) the parenteral route; that is, exposure to contaminated blood, including blood products, transfusions, occupational exposure, and sharing of needles; and (3) perinatally or across the placenta; that is, infected woman to fetus or exposure in utero, during birth, or to the infant via breastfeeding (ANA, 1988; CDC, 1987; & CDC, 1992).

Piemme and Bolle (1990) stated that since the onset of the AIDS epidemic, five groups have been identified at risk. They are as follows:

- sexually active homosexual and bisexual men with multiple sex partners

- present or past users of intravenous drugs

- patients who have been transfused with blood or blood products (prior to 1985 in the United States)

- heterosexual partners of persons with AIDS or of persons infected with HIV

- persons with hemophilia

Homosexual/bisexual men and intravenous drug users account for the majority of people with AIDS or HIV infection in the United States. Of alarming concern is the increasing number of heterosexual transmissions, especially among blacks and Hispanics. This in turn has resulted in an increased rate of HIV infection in women and children as well.

It has been found that blood, semen, and vaginal/cervical secretions contain sufficient concentrations of HIV to transmit the infection (Friedland & Klein, 1987). Transmission of HIV may take place when contact with semen occurs during sexual intercourse (vaginal and anal), oral sex (fellatio), and donor insemination. It may also be transmitted when there is exposure to vaginal/cervical secretions during vaginal intercourse and oral sex (cunnilingus). According to the Centers for Disease Control (CDC) (1992), in the United States, HIV is transmitted primarily through sexual contact.

A direct route for transmission of HIV includes the sharing of injection needles, syringes, and other drug-injection paraphernalia contaminated with blood containing HIV (CDC, 1992). Intravenous drug users that are infected with HIV can transmit the virus to their needle-sharing and/or sex partners. In pregnant women, it is transmitted to their offspring (Friedland & Klein, 1987).

Since mid-1985, all blood donations in the United States have been screened for HIV. Transfusions of whole blood, plasma, platelets, or blood cells have resulted in the transmission of HIV (Friedland & Klein, 1987). Although the screening procedures have decreased the number of transmissions via transfusions, it is believed that there will continue to be cases of AIDS identified because there is a long incubation period.

The incidence of HIV infection among hemophiliacs has also been investigated. Hemophiliacs are treated with the clotting factor derived from the pooled plasma of many donors. Before blood testing for HIV was implemented in 1985, the virus was transmitted to people with hemophilia through infusions of clotting factor concentrates (Friedland & Klein, 1987). The Centers for Disease Control estimate that the majority of those with hemophilia B have been infected with HIV (Stehr-Green, Holman, Jason & Evatt, 1988).

Incidence of AIDS among women has been and continues to be on the increase. Women infected with the HIV, even if asymptomatic, have the potential to transmit the virus perinatally. According to Oxtoby (1990), HIV infection can be passed from mothers to their offspring by three routes: in utero through the fetal-maternal circulation, by inoculation during labor and vaginal or cesarean delivery, and through infected breast milk after birth.

According to the CDC (1993), a few health care workers (HCW) have been infected with HIV through occupational exposure. The adherence to and use of universal precautions with all patients in the health care setting is the most prudent way to prevent occupational exposure. The use of universal precautions cannot be overemphasized since there is no sure way of identifying all those infected with HIV or other blood-borne pathogens. Universal precautions apply to blood, semen, vaginal secretions, cerebral fluid, synovial fluid, pleural fluid, peritoneal fluid, pericardial fluid, amniotic fluid, and any body fluid containing visible blood. Universal precautions do not apply to feces, nasal secretions, sputum, sweat, tears, urine, and vomitus unless they contain visible blood.

To prevent exposure to HIV infection, universal precautions must be observed from the first contact with *all* patients. Personal protective equipment (gown, gloves, goggles/face shield, and mask) should be used with direct patient care activities. Care must be taken to dispose of contaminated dressings and needles correctly. Strict sterilization guidelines must be followed for all reusable equipment for patient care (Porche, 1991).

The preceding information is alarming and is evidence that many populations are at risk for getting HIV infection or AIDS. It has been suggested that the best protection against HIV/AIDS is to adopt risk-free or low-risk behavior. Examples of risk-free or low-risk behaviors include abstinence or long-term mutually monogamous sexual relationships between two uninfected partners, use of condoms, avoiding drug use and the sharing of needles, and the practice of universal precautions by health care workers. These behaviors are essential to stopping the spread of HIV (Porth, 1994, p. 295).

NURSING AND AIDS

Grady (1989) described nursing as a profession with built-in risks. Throughout any given work day, a nurse may be at risk of exposure to radiation, stress, potential back injury, infectious diseases, and other threats to health (p. 526). Nurses traditionally have accepted the idea that some degree of personal risk is inherent in caring for the sick. This responsibility is based upon the obligation to give respectful, individualized care without discrimination (Reisman, 1988).

Throughout history, epidemics and disease have always played a major role in the human experience. While epidemics and disease create chaos and devastate the lives of many, they also bring people together to fight for the common good of all involved. Although some may react to a crisis with denial, fear, and even hatred, there are many who rise to the occasion to portray the best humanity has to offer: compassion and bravery in the face of the unknown (Meyer, 1991). Nurses are among those individuals who have always responded to help meet the needs arising because of a crisis.

Today, nurses continue to muster forces to fight what is the most devastating epidemic this generation has ever known: AIDS (Reisman, 1988). Never before has the profession of nursing been presented with such a challenge. Nurses in all types of health care agencies and in all clinical specialties face the complexities of giving care to HIV-infected individuals. According to Hicken (1990), "the challenge of HIV has presented the profession with the need to equip itself not only with the baseline knowledge of aetiology and the ways in which HIV can be transmitted, but also with an understanding of the psychosocial effects of HIV and AIDS" (p. 32).

The AIDS epidemic has brought many concerns, not only to the public, but to the profession of nursing as well. Because nurses are the health care professionals who are on the "front line" of providing care to patients with AIDS, they are being forced to examine and evaluate their own attitudes concerning a multitude of social taboos. According to Hicken (1990), nurses are faced with a multiplicity of issues that include loss, bereavement, sexuality, intravenous drug abuse, and alternate lifestyles.

Bolle (1988) identified specific factors related to AIDS that contribute to increased stress among caregivers. These include:

- fear of contagion
- issues in sexuality
- death and dying
- stigma
- exposure to alternate lifestyles
- issues of confidentiality (p. 844)

Fear of Contagion

Because of the contagious nature of AIDS, there has been much fear and anxiety felt by those providing care for these individuals. The following story depicts the feelings of a nurse and her fellow workers when one of their patients was diagnosed with AIDS.

What Is the Matter With Alexandro?

It is funny how people change when they hear something that they don't like. For example, before we knew Alexandro had AIDS we didn't think twice about touching him or being around him. Once we knew, though, our actions and thoughts about him were different. Before the diagnosis, we would take our time to talk with him, but now we were rushing to wash our hands. Poor man, we were sure he felt the cold-ness and the discrimination, but we couldn't help our feelings either.

Huerta and Oddi (1992) pointed out that findings from surveys of practicing nurses show that they harbor significant concerns about their personal safety (p. 221). According to Sullivan and Mills (1990), the risk of contraction in healthy nurses is extremely low, especially if common-sense precautions are used. They further stated that adherence to universal precautions is especially important in emergency settings and for patients with known AIDS infection, where the risk of body fluid exposure is dramatically increased (p. 13).

In order to face and overcome the fear of contagion, nurses must acquire the necessary knowledge and skills needed to care for patients with HIV/AIDS. Huerta and Oddi (1992) pointed out that if individual nurses are unable to fulfill their professional responsibilities to HIV/AIDS patients because of fear or a lack of requisite knowledge, they should rectify the situation as soon as possible or seek employment where HIV/AIDS patients are less likely to be encountered. Scherer, Haughy, and Wie, (1989) and Brennan (1988) agreed that perhaps deliberately seeking to care for these patients will help to conquer morbid fears; increased experience in providing care has been identified as a factor that may decrease the fear of contracting HIV/AIDS.

Issues of Sexuality

The issue of sexuality is often a major source of stress for health care providers because AIDS challenges the foundation of one's sexuality. Bolle (1988) believed that a distinction needs to be made between heterosexual and homosexual professionals. On the one hand, heterosexual nurses, whether male or female, may experience homophobia and feel very uncomfortable caring for homosexual persons with AIDS. These professionals may exhibit moralistic, punitive, or avoidance behavior toward the patient. They may be judgmental and condemn the patient and are therefore unable to understand the disease in its context.

On the other hand, the issue of sexuality becomes even more complex when it comes to homosexual nurses, especially homosexual male nurses. Bolle (1988) stated that openly homosexual nurses may be very much at risk for overidentification with AIDS patients. These nurses may overstep professional boundaries and become overinvolved with patients. Overidentification by these nurses may lead to an increased fear of coming down with the disease. This may result in exhibition of hypochondriacal reactions that may eventually have negative effects on job performance.

Nurses must explore their own feelings concerning sexuality. Acceptance of the patient as an individual needing the nurse's guidance and support is vital for establishing a therapeutic nurse-patient relationship.

Death and Dying

Daily confrontation with terminal illness is always a source of stress for the health care professional. The fact that AIDS has such a grim prognosis and that it affects primarily young and productive people makes it even harder. This exposure to death and dying may cause what Bolle (1988) called "bereavement overload." A nurse caring for patients with AIDS may experience both the physical and psychological signs and symptoms of grief and bereavement. Nurses who are motivated by a sense of duty to work with the dying AIDS patient need to be psychologically equipped. They need to be strong enough to meet the demands of working with these patients to prevent burnout.

Stigma

A stigma is a negative image or attitude placed on individuals who have violated society's taboos by becoming associated with areas viewed as forbidden (Goffman, 1963). AIDS is associated with two taboos in our society: illicit sex and drug abuse. The stigma associated with AIDS is of major concern to those involved with the care of these patients. AIDS is often associated with shame and disgrace. A nurse whose practice involves the care of patients with AIDS may be stigmatized by family members and friends who wonder what satisfaction could be obtained from caring for "those people" (Bolle, 1988).

Because of the stigma associated with a diagnosis of AIDS, parents are often unable to tell friends that their son died of AIDS. Homosexuals are afraid to admit to a diagnosis of AIDS and others are afraid to admit to a friendship with a person who has died of AIDS. Instead, they tell others "He had cancer" or "He died of pneumonia" or "I really did not know him very well." This inability to admit the truth of the death or the truth of the relationship can leave the bereaved angry, depressed, and extremely lonely.

Susan and George

Susan, a veteran nurse of over 15 years, stood by George when the doctor told him that he was HIV positive. Over the years, she had seen a lot and had met a lot of people, but there was something about George that really touched her. She noticed that he was always alone when he came to see the doctor. Susan asked George if his family knew about his condition. George informed her that they accepted the fact that he was gay, but had not wanted anything to do with him since he had been diagnosed with AIDS. He stated that they told him that he had brought it on himself.

Exposure to Alternate Lifestyles

For the first time in their professional life, nurses may be exposed to working with homosexuals and/or intravenous drug users (Bolle, 1988). If they are not prepared to work with these patients, then feelings of shock and disgust may surface. The following story tells of a nurse's first encounter with a patient who was an IV drug abuser.

Ralph and Linda

Ralph, a nurse working at a doctor's office, remembers the first time he met Linda. She was ill and frail looking. Linda was 25 years old and had come in complaining of a cough with bloody phlegm, chest pain, and very high fevers. Her x-ray revealed pneumocystis carinii pneumonia. She admitted that she was HIV positive and had contracted it through IV drug abuse. After that first encounter with Linda, Ralph felt somewhat perturbed by the situation. His emotions were in turmoil. He felt angry that this young woman, approximately the same age as he, had such a bleak future. What had made her do what she did? How could she do that to herself? To her family?

Occasionally, these feelings by the nurse exist because of conflicting individual, religious, or moral beliefs. The nurse's value system will be challenged because caring for AIDS patients means providing care to homosexuals, bisexuals, drug abusers, and/or drug addicts. A nurse with value conflicts needs to use value clarification to rationally approach the issues. This will help prevent value judgments from affecting the quality of care given to these individuals (Schietinger, 1986).

Confidentiality

The issue of confidentiality, according to the laws of ethics, involves protecting the patient's record with respect to the press, the family, and friends. The nurse is obligated to preserve the principle of confidentiality in the practice of nursing. This is founded in the patient's right to privacy and the preservation of the nurse-patient relationship (Reisman, 1988). At times, the nurse may feel pressure from outside sources to reveal privileged information about individuals and must be on guard for inquisitive telephone calls or suspicious visitors.

A major source of concern for the nurse regarding confidentiality may occur when the patient requests that family or friends not be told about the illness and disease. It is especially difficult when the nurse is not able to inform sexual partners who may be infected and at risk for infecting others.

Often the patient does not want family or friends to know about his lifestyle or the diagnosis of AIDS. The nurse is often caught between protecting the patient's right to privacy and the pressure of answering questions from well-meaning friends and family. Nurses need to carefully apply the principle of confidentiality and ethical guidelines to the practice of nursing (Reisman, 1988).

CARING FOR THE AIDS PATIENT

The care of the patient with AIDS can be characterized as difficult, personally demanding, and humbling (Carson & Green, 1992). This is often true because the process of dying as experienced by the AIDS patient is not a gentle one. The life of an AIDS patient is often characterized by repeated infections, debilitating diarrhea, wasting of once-robust bodies, intermittent but soaring fevers, unrelenting fatigue, disfiguring lesions, and sometimes dementia (Carson & Green, 1992, p. 210). Although our health care system focuses on cure, the finality of the diagnosis of patients with AIDS is a constant reminder that a cure is not an option. Acknowledgment of the fact that there is no curative treatment is necessary. Nurses who can admit this fact can shift priorities from curative measures to focus on the use of self to express acceptance and provide emotional support. The nurse's exploration of ways to improve quality, if not duration, of life for these patients will provide comfort for the patient and satisfaction for the nurse (Carson & Green, 1992). The focus of care may not be on healing the body of the AIDS patient, but on healing the spirit, fostering reconciliation, and bringing harmony to a troubled soul.

The nursing profession has responded to the epidemic with skill, expertise, and care for these patients. Nurses must continue to equip themselves with the knowledge and skills needed to provide palliative care. They need to nurture personal healing qualities to provide the best possible care to the patient with AIDS.

Nurses need to continue to work together to prevent burnout and promote quality patient care. Support groups for nurses involved in the care of AIDS patients are beneficial. These support groups provide the caregiver with opportunities to verbalize feelings, clarify values, and work through personal feelings of grief.

LOSS AND BEREAVEMENT DUE TO AIDS

By the time a person is diagnosed with AIDS, the individual may have already suffered the loss of family members, significant others, or friends to this disease. No matter the circumstances in which the person has acquired HIV/AIDS, the person may experience altered social roles, fear of discrimination in the workplace, and even loss of employment because of the disease. This is a stressful time for the individual. In some cases, the individual facing the death of someone close to him may also be facing the possibility of his own death as well. This is a difficult situation to be facing and at times can be overwhelming.

Another disturbing facet is the anticipation of becoming progressively disabled because of the deterioration of physical and cognitive abilities resulting from AIDS. The prospect of mental and physical deterioration can be extremely frightening and depressing for the individual.

The initial stage of diagnosis is characterized by a variety of complex reactions that often vacillate between fear, grief, guilt, anger, uncertainty, and sometimes hope. The emotional upheaval experienced is related to the degree of severity and progression of the disease in each individual. On good days, the person with AIDS may feel fine and look forward to being with loved ones. At other times, the thought of becoming incapacitated or of experiencing a traumatic death may be overwhelming (Piemme & Bolle, 1990).

Besides the fear associated with living and dying with AIDS, feelings of rejection, discrimination, and isolation also come into play. These negative feelings often surface in coworkers, friends, and family members, resulting in the patient experiencing major changes in social roles. Individuals with AIDS may no longer be unconditionally accepted by people around them or by society. Maintaining fulfilling relationships becomes an extremely difficult if not impossible task to accomplish. Rubinow (1984) reported that AIDS patients had to deal with a loss of social support manifested by abandonment of family and friends. This loss occurred at a time when the need for support from loved ones was imperative. In a study conducted by Durham and Hatcher (1984), they observed the lack of support systems in these patients and concluded that this was a result of the patient's "having maintained a lifestyle that alienated his family or having been unsuccessful in establishing an enduring, meaningful relationship with another person" (p. 302). Moreover, once a diagnosis of AIDS was confirmed, these patients experienced more fragmentation in support systems because of the stigma and fears associated with the disease.

AIDS usually affects those in the most active years of life. The vibrancy that is typically associated with the young and middle adult years is challenged by the possibility of repeated infections, neurological impairment, and apathy (Piemme & Bolle, 1990). These, along with the changes that occur in the patient's physical stamina and general appearance, will have a major affect on identity and self-esteem. The fear of social isolation and abandonment can be of major concern to the AIDS patient (Christ & Wiener, 1985).

The losses experienced by a person with AIDS will be many. From the moment of the diagnosis, grief over the loss of health, family, finances, and friends, and grief over the loss of one's own life will permeate the person's daily life. Nothing will ever be the same again. There will be no opportunity for a second chance. Unfortunately, for many this is also a time of desolation and fear of facing death alone.

Several theories of bereavement were introduced in previous chapters. These theories are applicable to any individual who has suffered the loss of a loved one. There still remains a substantial lack of support and understanding toward the grief associated with the loss of a loved one to AIDS. Ferrell and Boyle (1992) pointed out that "given the present societal norms, persons dying from AIDS face a stigmatized death while surviving partners, particularly those in homosexual relationships, may experience a stigmatized grief" (p. 127).

Survivors of persons dying from AIDS are a new population of grievers experiencing common grief reactions. In AIDS-related grieving, there are several concerns that may compound the problems facing the bereaved individual. One major concern for the bereaved individual is the fear of developing the disease by virtue of the previous relationship. The person who has been engaged in a sexual relationship with the deceased has to deal with the stigma associated with this disease (Helgadottir, 1990). Factors contributing to the stigma associated with AIDS include fear, prejudice, and ignorance. The stigma leads the bereaved toward social isolation, intense fear, and difficulty in forming new relationships. The fear and isolation the bereaved individual experiences becomes a constant reminder that reinforces identification with the deceased.

Bereaved individuals may choose not to be tested for HIV antibodies because of the fear of having the disease confirmed by the test (Helgadottir, 1990). Making this choice may further intensify the apprehension and stress over the situation. For some, refusal to be tested is an effective coping mechanism, while for others it is a continuous source of worry. By not knowing whether the infection is present or not, the individual postpones facing the prospect of having to fight AIDS without the support of the deceased (Helgadottir, 1990).

Because the individual may choose to deny the fact that the HIV infection may be present, reentering the social scene and establishing other meaningful relationships is often difficult. The fear of becoming infected or infecting someone else is a reality that must be faced. The fear felt by these individuals is often accompanied by feelings of guilt. This guilt is due in part to suspecting or perhaps knowing that they may have infected their partner, spouse, or child.

The reality for the bereaved individual includes facing the fact that his source of emotional support may no longer exist. This reality and the lack of support from family and friends because of the stigma associated with the disease can also contribute to unresolved grief by the bereaved individual. Outside support may not be sought for fear of being rejected because the grief is associated with an AIDS-related death (Ferrel & Boyle, 1992). Keeping the deceased person's sexual orientation, IV drug abuse, and AIDS diagnosis a secret can hamper the resolution of the grief and compound the agony felt by the bereaved (Murphy & Perry, 1988).

The bereaved must face and deal with many concerns that will arise from the death of the loved one. All these concerns can be detrimental to the ability of the bereaved to successfully complete the grieving process. In fact, the bereaved individual who has lost a loved one to AIDS is considered at high risk for complicated grieving. If the griever was involved in a homosexual relationship, the fear of developing AIDS, the stigma associated with the diagnosis, and lack of support from those around him must be faced.

One of the hardest things bereaved individuals must face is not only the death of their loved one, but their own mortality as well. This may be the most difficult task these individuals have to face. Mentally, physically, and emotionally they may not be prepared to face the task of contemplating death, especially their own.

COPING WITH THE LOSS DUE TO AIDS

Coping with death and dying or loss and bereavement is never easy. When death is laced with fear, prejudice, and stigma, dealing with the loss of a loved one is made even harder. There is no one way to help the bereaved individual cope with the grief of losing someone to AIDS and all the complications associated with the loss. The individual's coping mechanisms will be tried to the limits. Eventually, the survival of the bereaved will depend on the strengths of the individual's coping abilities.

If the bereaved was involved in a homosexual relationship, the death must often be faced without the usual understanding and support from family and friends. This lack of support may force the bereaved to suppress the grief process resulting in perpetuation of grief or complete denial of the death. Not being able to openly grieve over a loved one can result in the person experiencing increased levels of anxiety and depression.

Helping the bereaved individual cope with the death of a loved one due to AIDS will require the utmost caring, understanding, and support from those involved with the situation. Jones (1988) believed that nurses have a "unique opportunity to become agents of change and act as patients' advocates and participate in a pioneering approach to care" (p. 57). He feels that nurses can facilitate effective preparatory grief work by fostering an atmosphere in which the homosexual couple is allowed to react within the context of their relationship. This will allow the individuals to openly share their concerns and feelings, and to effectively begin grief work.

Nurses are also in a position to identify those at risk for complicated grieving. By identifying those at risk early in a given situation, referrals to appropriate sources for support can be made. Whatever the individual's beliefs may be, nurses can help make the connection needed for continued help (Garrett, 1988). Proper support will help meet the emotional needs of the bereaved and help them through the grieving process.

The nurse who seeks to help the individual with this type of grief faces a formidable task. Healing strategies such as journal writing, relaxation techniques, volunteering to serve on local AIDS councils, reaching out to others, or attending a support group may provide comfort to the bereaved. These healing strategies are explored further in chapter 9.

The homosexual community has rallied to provide support to the AIDS patient and to those who grieve because of losing someone to AIDS. Without the benefit of a support group specifically for these individuals, grieving may be difficult. A support group for the bereaved can provide a nonthreatening environment in which to express feelings and talk with others who share similar experiences. These groups may be lead by nurses, clinical nurse specialists, psychiatric nurse practitioners, or others who have suffered a similar loss.

SUMMARY

Death and bereavement are issues that continually challenge our values and beliefs. Death and bereavement due to AIDS are issues that present further challenges in an area where attitudes are firmly entrenched (Jones, 1988). According to Callanan and Kelly (1992), we need to "recall the emotional stages of dealing with death—denial, anger, bargaining, depression, acceptance— and remember that these feelings arise as the dying person and others involved struggle to come to terms with the reality of the diagnosis, adjusting to life with this illness, and preparing for approaching death" (p. 240). As nurses, we need to address these issues to provide effective and compassionate care to those in need and recognize that both the psychological and the physical needs must be met (Jones, 1988). In meeting these needs, nurses can provide the most appropriate care possible to foster true dignity in death and facilitate bereavement.

RESOURCES

If you have questions about HIV or AIDS, you can call:

- American Foundation for AIDS Research
  1-213-857-5900

- Gay Men's Health Crisis
  1-212-807-6655

- National AIDS Hotline
  1-800-342-2437
  1-800-344-7432 (Spanish)
  1-800-243-7889 (for the hearing-impaired)

- National AIDS Information Clearinghouse
  1-800-458-5231

- San Francisco AIDS Foundation
  1-415-863-2437

REFLECTIONS

1. What are your feelings concerning alternate lifestyles? Homosexuality? Illicit drug use?

2. Have you provided care for an HIV positive or AIDS patient? How did you feel or how would you feel about providing care for an HIV/AIDS patient?

3. Has the information provided in this chapter made a difference to your way of thinking regarding the needs of the person with AIDS? Your role as caregiver?

References

American Nurses' Association. (1988). Nursing and the human immunodeficiency virus: A guide for nursings' response to AIDS. In P. G. Beare & J. Myers (Eds.), *Principles and practices of adult health nursing* (p. 1029). St. Louis: Mosby.

Bolle, J. L. (1988). Supporting the deliverers of care: Strategies to support nurses and prevent burnout. *Nursing Clinics of North America, 23*(4), 843–849.

Brennan, L. (1988). The battle against AIDS. *Nursing, 18*(4), 60–64.

Burris, S., Dalton, H. L., Miller, J. L., & the Yale AIDS Law Project (Eds.). (1993). *AIDS law today: A new guide for the public.* New Haven, CT: Yale University Press.

Callanan, M., & Kelly, P. (1992). *Final gifts.* New York: Bantam Books.

Carson, V. B., & Green, H. (1992). Spiritual well-being: A predictor of hardiness in patients with acquired immunodeficiency syndrome. *Journal of Professional Nursing, 8*(4), 209–220.

Centers for Disease Control. (1987). Recommendation for prevention of HIV transmission in health-care settings. In P. G. Beare & J. Myers (Eds.), *Principles and practices of adult health nursing* (p. 1029). St. Louis: Mosby.

Centers for Disease Control. (1992). HIV/AIDS surveillance report. In P. G. Beare & J. Myers (Eds.), *Principles and practices of adult health nursing* (p. 1029). St. Louis: Mosby.

Centers for Disease Control. (1992). Mortality patterns in the United States, 1989. In C. M. Porth, *Pathophysiology: Concepts of altered health states* (pp. 283–286). Philadelphia: J. B. Lippincott Co.

Centers for Disease Control. (1993). 1993 revised classification system for HIV infection and expanded surveillance case definition for AIDS among adolescents and adults. In P. G. Beare & J. Myers (Eds.), *Principles and practices of adult health nursing* (p. 1029). St. Louis: Mosby.

Centers for Disease Control. (1993). HIV/AIDS surveillance report. In C. M. Porth, *Pathophysiology: Concepts of altered health states* (pp. 283–286). Philadelphia: J. B. Lippincott Co.

Christ, G. H., & Wiener, L. S. (1985). Psychosocial issues in AIDS. In V.T. De Vita, S. Hellman, & S. A. Rosenberg (Eds.), *AIDS: Etiology, diagnosis, treatment and prevention* (pp. 275–297). Philadelphia: J. B. Lippincott.

Curran, J. W., Morgan, W. M., Hardy, A. M., Jaffe, H. W., Darrow, W. W., & Dowdle, W. R. (1985). The epidemiology of AIDS: Current status and future prospects. In C. M. Porth, *Pathophysiology: Concepts of altered health states* (pp. 283–286). Philadelphia: J. B. Lippincott Co.

Durham, J. D., & Hatcher, B. (1984). Reducing psychological complications for the critically ill AIDS patient. *Dimensions in Critical Care Nursing, 3*, 301–306.

Ferrell, J. A., & Boyle, J. S. (1992). Bereavement experiences: Caring for a partner with AIDS. *Journal of Community Health Nursing, 9*(3), 127–135.

Flaskerud, J. H. (Ed.). (1989). *AIDS/HIV infection: A reference guide for nursing professionals.* Philadelphia: W. B. Saunders.

Friedland, G., & Klein, S. (1987). Transmission of the human immunodeficiency virus. In C. M. Porth, *Pathophysiology: Concepts of altered health states* (pp. 283–286). Philadelphia: J. B. Lippincott Company.

Garrett, J. E. (1988). The AIDS patient: Helping him and his parents cope. *Nursing 88, 88*, 50–52.

Goffman, E. (1963). *Stigma.* Englewood Cliffs, NJ: Prentice Hall.

Grady, C. (1989). Ethical issues in providing nursing care to human immunodeficiency virus-infected populations. *Nursing Clinics of North America, 24*(2), 523–534.

Helgadottir, H. (1990). AIDS: Grieving alone. *Nursing Times, 86*(37), 28–32.

Hicken, I. (1990). AIDS: Taking the education initiative. *Nursing Times, 86*(37), 32–35.

Huerta, S. R., & Oddi, L. F. (1992). Refusal to care for patients with human immunodeficiency virus/acquired immunodeficiency syndrome: Issues and responses. *Journal of Professional Nursing, 8*(4), 221–230.

Jones, A. (1988). Nothing gay about bereavement. *Nursing Times, 8*(84), 55–57.

Meyer, C. (1991). Nursing and AIDS: A decade of caring. *American Journal of Nursing, 91*(12), 26–31.

Murphy, P., & Perry, K. (1988). Hidden grievers. *Death Studies, 12*, 451–462.

Nuland, S. B. (1994). *How we die: Reflections on life's final chapter.* New York: Alfred A. Knopf.

Oxtoby, M. J. (1990). Perinatally acquired human immunodeficiency virus infection. In C. M. Porth, *Pathophysiology: Concepts of altered health states* (p. 285). Philadelphia: J. B. Lippincott Co.

Piemme, J. A., & Bolle, J. L. (1990). Coping with grief in response to caring for persons with AIDS. *The American Journal of Occupational Therapy, 44,* 266–269.

Porche, D. J. (1991). Universal precautions. In P. G. Beare & J. Myers (Eds.), *Principles and practices of adult health nursing* (p. 1039). St. Louis: Mosby.

Porth, C. M. (1994). *Pathophysiology: Concepts of altered health states.* Philadelphia: J. B. Lippincott Co.

Reisman, E. C. (1988). Ethical issues confronting nursing. *Nursing Clinics of North America, 23*(4), 789–801.

Rubinow, D. R. (1984). The psychology impact of AIDS. *Topics in Clinical Nursing, 6,* 26–30.

Scherer, Y. K., Haughy, B. P., & Wie, Y. B. (1989). AIDS: What are nurses' concerns? *Clinical Nurse Specialist, 3*(1), 4–54.

Schietinger, H. (1986). A home care plan for AIDS. *American Journal of Nursing, 86,* 1021–1028.

Stehr-Green, J., Holman, R., Jason, J., & Evatt, B. (1988). Hemophilia-associated AIDS in the United States, 1981 to September, 1987. *American Journal of Public Health, 78,* 439–442.

Sullivan, P. A., & Mills, M. E., (1990). Policy considerations related to AIDS. *Journal of Nursing Administration, 20*(1), 12–18.

Ungvarski, P. J., & Schmidt, J. (1992, November). AIDS patients under attack. *RN,* 36–45.

RESPONSE TO THE TRAUMATIC DEATH OF A LOVED ONE

7

Sally S. Roach

The two sidedness of death is a fundamental feature of death . . . The sting of death is less sharp for the person who dies than it is for the bereaved survivor . . . There are two parties to the suffering that death inflicts; and in the apportionment of this suffering, the survivor takes the brunt.

Arnold Toynbee

INTRODUCTION

Facing the death of a loved one is a traumatic and painful experience whatever the circumstances. With expected or anticipated death, the survivor has time to prepare for the loss. There is time to reconcile conflicts within relationships. There is time to explore thoughts of the future without the loved one. Words necessary for closure may be spoken. Simply having the time to say "I love you" or "Good-bye" can provide a measure of comfort.

When death occurs suddenly or as the result of a trauma, there is no time for closure. The relationship is abruptly and permanently severed. While sudden or traumatic death does not necessarily cause greater pain to the survivor, the shock is so strong that adaptation becomes more difficult (Lightner & Hathaway,

1990). Even with anticipated death, we are never totally prepared for the loss of a loved one. When death is imminent, the survivor analyzes every detail of the loved one's condition, hoping for some sign of recovery. Friends and family members are often unable to face the certainty of death. The pain is too great to let go. Bob discusses his shock and pain at the loss of his brother, although intellectually he knew that death was near.

Dave's Death

When my brother Dave died, Julie, his daughter, and I were with him. I had prayed fervently for Dave's healing. As he became worse I thought, "God can still raise him up from his sick bed, so I can't give up." The hospice nurse had diligently told us that death was coming, but I resented it. I fought it. When death finally seemed inevitable, I gave in. I had read that the dying sometimes need the assurance of loved ones that it is okay to go. Julie and I started telling him, "It's all right Daddy, you can go," "It's all right Dave, you can go." Both Julie and I were crying, watching as he struggled to breathe. Julie asked if he could hear us. Dave turned his head toward her, gave one positive nod and took one last breath. Although I knew death was near, the shock was overpowering. I cannot keep from crying even now, as I remember these events, over a year after his death.

Although Dave's death was anticipated, his brother was shocked at its occurrence. This is a normal response to the trauma of the death of a loved one. After the initial shock and dismay, most grievers continue through the grieving process without exhibiting the symptoms associated with complicated grief.

A sudden, unexpected, or violent death can greatly intensify and complicate the grieving process. The remainder of this chapter focuses on the grief that occurs due to the loss of a loved one from a death due to traumatic circumstances, such as a homicide, a suicide, or accidental death.

TRAUMATIC DEATH DEFINED

Figley (1985, p. xviii) defined the grief associated with traumatic death as "an emotional state of discomfort and stress resulting from memories of an extraordinary, catastrophic experience which shattered the survivor's sense of invulnerability to harm." The survivor is thrown into a state of extreme disequilibrium caused by this catastrophic occurrence. This disequilibrium results in feelings of powerlessness and vulnerability which can lead to complications in the grieving process and in recovery. Therese A. Rando (1993), a leading authority on traumatic death, identified situations that help classify a death or circumstance as traumatic:

- death that occurs suddenly
- death as a result of violence
- death viewed as preventable
- multiple deaths
- a personal threat to one's own survival
- witnessing the traumatic death of another

Any sudden, unanticipated death, or any death where violence plays a part increases the risk for complicated mourning (Rando, 1993).

COMPLICATED GRIEF

Complicated mourning is difficult to define. According to Wolfelt (1991), the difference between normal and complicated mourning is related to the intensity and duration of a specific response. Therefore, the presence or absence of any specific grief response does not necessarily contribute to the difference between normal and pathological grief. Welue (1975) suggested the following criteria be used to identify complicated grief: evidence of self-destructive behavior; presence of physiological problems; social withdrawal; depression; and hospitalization for psychiatric symptoms. When these symptoms persist and/or increase in severity, complicated grief is a possibility. According to Harowitz, Bonanno, and Holen (1993), in complicated grief, aspects of normal grief become exaggerated or distorted. For example, numbness is exaggerated to a point where the survivor is unable to feel any emotion or even a sense of self. Denial persists for longer periods and anger becomes extreme. Excessive drinking or drug abuse may become a major coping mechanism. Extreme social withdrawal may occur as evidenced by failure to hold a job, inability to develop any meaningful relationships or antisocial behavior. In complicated mourning, there is a failure to give up the lost loved one and an inability to reinvest in life. This results in a stagnation in the grieving process and prevents resolution of grief. Grief that lasts over 2 years, the lack of any expression of grief, or the presence of exaggerated responses to grief suggest pathology. These manifestations indicate the need for further assessment and possible intervention by a psychiatrist or a psychiatric clinical nurse specialist.

Classifications of Complicated Grief

Wolfelt (1991) subdivided complicated grief into four classifications: chronic grief, distorted grief, converted grief, and absent grief. An understanding of these four classifications can help the nurse in understanding the different aspects of complicated grief. The following descriptions incorporate Wolfelt's (1991) observations concerning complicated grief.

Chronic Grief   This form of grief persists over an extended period (2 years or more). Like John, in chronic grief, the griever is unable to relinquish the lost loved one and reinvest in life.

Chronic Grief

John, age 66, is a retired retailer. John's daughter and her fiancé were killed in an automobile accident when returning to the local university after a holiday. Although this event occurred 18 years ago, John frequently mentions his daughter during conversation with others. He weeps and tells of the tragedy as if it were a recent occurrence. His inability to accept the loss and sadness over the event are evident although many years have passed.

In chronic grief, the griever's continued focus on the deceased leads to chronic depression and deep sadness.

Distorted Grief   This type of grief can occur at any point in the grieving process. The griever develops a preoccupation with one area and cannot progress through the stages of grief. The emotions most frequently causing stagnation in the grieving process are guilt and anger (Wolfelt, 1991). In Dorothy's case her preoccupation with guilt over the death of her daughter interfered with the relationship with her daughter who was still alive.

Dorothy's Guilt

Twins Julie and Juliet, 8 years old, begged to cross the street to the local convenience store. Their mother, Dorothy, at first denied their eager request. Later, she relented and allowed the children to go, cautioning them to be very careful. When the twins arrived at the store, Julie needed more money for her purchases. She quickly turned to run back across the street to get more money from her mother. Her steps led her directly into the path of an oncoming car and instant death. Dorothy was completely devastated. She experienced extreme sadness and relentless pangs of guilt. Several years passed, but Dorothy continued to blame herself. So great was her guilt that she progressively withdrew from her surviving daughter.

Converted Grief   Converted grief is similar to a conversion reaction. To ease the pain of grief, the emotional pain is transferred to physical complaints. Jose Munoz's grief over the death of his wife was "converted" to physical complaints.

Converted Grief

Jose's wife had recently died of cancer of the colon. Jose loved his wife deeply, but was not able to grieve openly. Although Jose had always been in good health, he began to develop many physical complaints. Soon he was spending many hours in the doctor's office trying to find a reason for his pain. Many physical examinations failed to reveal any medical reason for his complaints.

Unfortunately Jose's physical complaints will probably continue until he deals with the emotional pain of his wife's death.

Absent Grief   In absent grief, the survivor remains in a continual state of denial. No feelings of grief are expressed because as emotions begin to surface, the survivor represses them so that the pain of the loss will be avoided. This inability to express the emotions of grief can lead to great inner turmoil. Mr. Grant lost his wife several years ago. However, if you met Mr. Grant, you would never suspect his wife was dead.

Mrs. Grant's Absence

By the way Mr. Grant speaks of his wife, some of his colleagues at the university where he teaches think that Mrs. Grant is very much alive. He speaks of her in the present tense. Mr. Grant lives alone in the same house that he and his wife occupied. Very little around the house has changed in the years since her death. Mrs. Grant's bedroom is still the same. Her clothes, although now outdated, are still in the closet. When asked about Mrs. Grant, Mr. Grant shrugs his shoulders and mumbles a vague excuse. Mr. Grant has been unable to accept the death of his wife and is living in a constant state of denial.

A variation of absent grief occurs when the survivor continues with life, never mentioning the deceased at all. All reminders of the deceased are removed and actions are as if the deceased never existed. Grief is absent because the loss has never been acknowledged.

DEATH BY VIOLENCE

Violence is becoming increasingly evident in today's society. More and more people are falling victim to its prey. Survivors who have lost loved ones through violence have a multiplicity of feelings, including shock, anxiety, terror, powerlessness, vulnerability, and victimization (Rando, 1994). These feelings lead to anger, guilt, and shame which predispose the survivor to complicated grief.

Anger

The anger associated with this type of grief is usually directed at the perpetrators of the violence and can lead to the desire for revenge. The survivor may become actively involved in seeking prosecution and/or obtaining restitution. Dealing with lawyers, court dates, and the trial can provide an outlet for anger (Lightner & Hathaway, 1990). Unfortunately, this type of activity can also delay grief. Preoccupation with seeking justice can place feelings on hold, allowing the survivor to procrastinate dealing with the pain of loss. Jean became so obsessed with obtaining justice for her son's death that grief was delayed. Jean's loss is portrayed in the following vignette.

Feeling the Loss

Thirty-nine-year-old Don was shot in his home by 2 armed intruders. Don returned fire. Although he wounded one of the intruders, they escaped. Don staggered from his house to his nearest neighbor, about ¼ mile away. He pounded on the door for help. He was unable to call out because of a bullet wound to the throat. The neighbor helped him to lie down and called for help, but Don died within a few minutes.

Today, Don's mother, Jean, has still shed no tears. Her heart is heavy, but she is unable to grieve. Instead she spends her days seeking to bring those who murdered her son to trial, wanting to see justice. Every day she goes and sits across the road from a little store where she feels those who know who killed her son work. She states, "I go there every day at 6:00 in the afternoon and just sit and pray. I pray Don's murderers will be brought to justice. That he can finally rest in peace. Maybe then I can weep, maybe then I can feel something besides this terrible anger." Today, 3 years later, Jean still waits. She waits for justice. She waits to grieve.

Guilt

Guilt and self-blame are also prominent feelings associated with traumatic death. These emotions are felt for a variety of reasons. Guilt over the inability to intervene during the incident is a common emotion. The griever may blame herself because of the inability to protect the loved one. Guilt over something that should have been done, but was not done, can intensify the grief. Survivors must be assisted to explore, understand, and redefine the feelings associated with survival guilt. Forgiveness of self or others may become a necessary part of healing.

Traumatic Imagery

In a study on bereavement after homicide, Rynearson and McCleery (1993) found that survivors whose loved ones died a violent death suffered "traumatic imagery." Traumatic imagery consists of vivid flashbacks and intense dreams in which the crime is reenacted in the mind of the survivor. These flashbacks occurred although the crime was seldom witnessed by the survivor. According to Rynearson and McCleery (1993), the flashbacks are so painful that survivors go to great lengths to avoid any cues that will result in an episode. They may avoid watching violent television shows or news reports containing violence. These flashbacks can occur up to several times a day and cause severe anxiety.

Additionally, the survivor may continuously relive the imagined feelings of terror and pain that the victim felt before death (Rynearson and McCleery, 1993). The reliving of the victim's terror, coupled with traumatic imagery and intense grief can lead to Post Traumatic Stress Disorder (PTSD).

Post Traumatic Stress Disorder

According to the American Psychiatric Association's *Diagnostic and Statistical Manual of Mental Disorders* (1994), PTSD may occur following any psychologically traumatic event that is outside the range of usual experience. The individual's response to the experience must involve intense fear, helplessness, or horror. The survivor persistently reexperiences the stimuli associated with the trauma. Any reminders of the event are tenaciously avoided. For PTSD to be diagnosed, the complete clinical picture must be present for longer than 1 month. The individual must also exhibit impairment in important areas of functioning such as those relating to social or occupational activities. For a complete clinical picture the reader is referred to the *Diagnostic and Statistical Manual of Mental Disorders* 4th ed.

PTSD is associated with veterans of the Vietnam War who have been unable to resolve the emotions of the traumatic experiences they endured during their war years. After returning from the war, they were unable to assume a normal lifestyle and suffered a wide range of symptoms. Symptoms of PTSD include:

- numbing of one's emotions
- recurrent dreams or nightmares related to the incident
- avoidance of thoughts and/or feelings associated with the event
- intense irritability or anger
- difficulty concentrating
- psychological distress to cues that symbolize or resemble the event, such as the anniversary of the trauma

- impaired interpersonal relationships (feeling detached or estranged)
- physiological complaints (peptic ulcer, migraine headaches, hypertension, bronchial asthma)
- sleep disturbances

Grieving after the loss of a loved one is a normal and necessary experience. However, a sudden, unexpected, or violent death may result in the survivor becoming so traumatized that symptoms associated with PTSD emerge. The terror-filled memories of survivors are comparable to the traumatic imagery experienced by survivors of the Vietnam War. Those mourning the traumatic death of a loved one do not automatically experience PTSD, but the possibility of PTSD exists and nurses must be aware of this possibility.

SUICIDE

Suicide is the voluntary and intentional destruction of oneself. In times past, suicide was considered a felony and was punished by a disgraceful burial and forfeiture of property (O'Hara, 1970). While laws no longer view suicide as a criminal offense, society often continues to stigmatize this type of death. Some religions persist in the belief that suicide is the ultimate sin and can only be rewarded by eternal punishment.

Guilt and Anger

The loss of a loved one from suicide is totally foreign and almost unthinkable to most people. Therefore, if suicide occurs, the survivor somehow feels to blame (Dunn & Morrish-Vidners, 1987–88). The survivor feels as if he has somehow failed his loved one.

Self-blame emerges because of perceptions by the survivor that he failed to notice clues of the impending suicide. Obscure clues such as giving away a valued object may have gone unheeded. The survivor feels guilt because of a failure to identify these clues before the suicide. In the survivor's mind, if these clues had been identified, the tragedy may have been prevented.

By failing to identify the clues, the survivor feels that he in some way contributed to the death. Self-blame may occur because the survivor feels he failed to provide adequate love and support to the loved one. This self-inflicted incrimination can cause the survivor much pain and self-reproach. These feelings of blame and self-reproach can lead to the "If only" syndrome.

"If only

I had tried harder to help . . .

I had paid more attention . . .

then maybe I could have prevented the suicide." These thoughts can plague the survivor and increase the pain.

Guilt and self-blame can turn to anger and another form of the "If only" syndrome develops.

"If only

you had come to me . . .

you had called me on the phone . . .

you had let me help you . . .

then maybe I could have prevented you from killing yourself." Intense anger is directed at the deceased for not seeking the help of the survivor or for making the choice to escape the problems of life through death.

The use of the "If only" syndrome gives the survivor someone besides herself to blame. This temporarily eases the pain and displaces the guilt. Eventually, however, the death must be faced realistically. These two conflicting emotions, guilt and anger, ebb and flow as the survivor attempts to come to terms with the death. The following vignette illustrates the feelings of guilt and anger in the mind of a young woman whose sister committed suicide.

The Death of Leah's Sister

Leah had just come in from a pleasant night with her older sister. The sisters were celebrating the end of Leah's first semester as a nursing student. The young women had spent the evening talking

and laughing. As Leah dressed for bed, she heard the deafening roar
of a gun. She quickly ran into her sister's room. There she found her
sister lying in a pool of blood, a gun at her side. Leah was hysterical.
How could this have happened? Why? She and her sister had enjoyed
such a good evening. All kinds of questions kept going through
Leah's mind, but there were no answers. Leah went through the
funeral in a daze. People were kind but distant, almost as if they did
not want to talk about what had happened. When classes started
again, Leah was unable to concentrate. Her grades were failing. Out
of desperation, Leah made an appointment to talk with one of her
nursing instructors. At first it was difficult, but soon she was weeping
uncontrollably. The instructor suggested they meet weekly. Together
they explored Leah's relationship with her sister. With time, Leah
released the anger at her sister and relinquished the guilt she felt for
not "seeing the clues" her sister was giving before the suicide. Leah
wrote a letter to her sister and visited her sister's grave. Leah made
peace with herself and her sister. The instructor also taught Leah
some simple relaxation techniques that helped her reduce stress.
Within several months, Leah's grades improved and she was eagerly
anticipating the beginning of her second year in nursing school.

Shame

Shame may also be experienced when a loved one takes his own
life (Calhoun, Selby, & Selby, 1982). There is a social stigma
attached to death by suicide. Dunn and Morrish-Vidners
(1987–88) reported that survivors of those who committed suicide
felt shame over the incident. These individuals used words such
as *embarrassed, awkward, ashamed,* and *afraid* when describing
their feelings when discussing the suicide with others. Societal
attitudes add to the guilt and shame of the survivor.

   Suicide is viewed by some as a failure of families to provide
the emotional support and caring necessary for the individual to
feel valued and loved. Family members feel ashamed that their

loved one was not strong enough to overcome the suicidal ideation or they feel ashamed that they were not able to help the loved one overcome the problems that led to the suicide. Shame leads to withdrawal and failure to discuss the circumstances of the death with others.

Survivor Support

Those who lose friends and loved ones to suicide receive less emotional support during grief than those who lose loved ones from natural death (Faberow, Gallagher, Thompson, Gilewski, & Thompson, 1992). Families may be unable to cope with the social stigma of suicide and repress their feelings, thereby increasing the possibility of complicated mourning. The nurse must be aware of the need for the survivors to have someone with which to discuss their emotions and feelings. Discussions of feelings and emotions are necessary for healing to begin. Survivor support groups or family therapy may be beneficial in releasing the pent-up feelings.

ACCIDENTAL DEATH

Another form of traumatic death is accidental death. Accidental death occurs from automobiles, knives, firearms, falls, drowning, natural disasters, and a multiplicity of other sources too many to name. Accidental deaths are difficult because of the sheer shock sustained from the unexpectedness of the death and the sense of preventability associated with the term "accident."

Preventability

Rando (1994) identified the issue of preventability as an area of concern in accidental death. When an event is viewed as preventable, the survivor is haunted with powerful feelings that the death did not have to occur. It could have been prevented. Much time and effort is spent searching for an explanation for the cause or reason for the death. Importance is placed on attaching responsibility and assigning blame for the accident (Rando, 1994). This searching is an effort to find meaning and regain a feeling of control over one's life.

Anger

Anger may also be directed at the one deemed responsible. Intense anger can cause the grieving process to stagnate and the griever can drown in the pain of grief.

The sense of injustice and the anger evoked from that injustice spurs the griever to action to dispel the pain. Activity can provide an outlet for the expression of the anger associated with grief. The griever can find solace in becoming actively involved in volunteer work or community service. She can give programs on teaching self-defense techniques, speak on the perils of alcohol, or become a gun control activist.

These activities can provide the survivor with ways to create meaning for the death. For example, teaching another woman to defend herself against an attacker may in some way help the survivor feel the death of her loved one was not in vain. The survivor crusading against driving while intoxicated feels that to keep one drunk off the road may save the life of another person's loved one. Too much involvement or too intense involvement can cause the grieving process to stagnate and the griever to become fixed in a sea of avoidance. Candi Lightner (1990) discussed the death of her daughter, Cari, as a result of an automobile accident involving a drunken driver. Anger was directed at the injustice of the judicial system. This system allowed an individual with four prior arrests to be out of jail on bond. The last arrest was only two days before her daughter's death. This injustice inspired Lightner to action.

Her anger and sense of helplessness led her to establish the organization, Mothers Against Drunk Drivers (MADD). Lightner spent the first several years after her daughter's death avoiding her grief through 24-hour days working with MADD. She stated "I was afraid to stop even for a moment, because I imagined that if I did I would drown in my grief" (Lightner & Hathaway, 1990, p. 11). Her activity in MADD became a way to escape facing the fact that her precious daughter was dead.

Healing did not begin for Lightner until she left MADD and allowed herself to actively grieve. Only when she began to nurture herself and allow the feelings of hurt and pain to be fully expressed did the sense of peace she so desperately needed emerge.

HEALING THE PAIN OF TRAUMATIC DEATH

As was previously discussed, losing a loved one as the result of traumatic death predisposes the survivor to complicated grief. Not only must the survivor deal with the pain of losing a loved one, but a totally unfathomable event has occurred that places the survivor in total disarray. The sheer unexpectedness of traumatic death leaves the survivor void of normal coping mechanisms due to the intensity of the shock. The nurse-healer must understand the implications of traumatic death and be alert for the possibility of complicated grief. Rando (1993) identified several factors innate in sudden, unanticipated death. These factors are important for the nurse-healer to consider when working with those who have lost loved ones from sudden death. Factors identified by Rando (1993) as influencing an individual's ability to cope with traumatic death include:

- The person's usual coping mechanisms are less effective due to the extreme shock of the death.

- The belief that the world is predictable and safe is destroyed, leaving the survivor with no confidence in his environment. This increases anxiety.

- Feelings of powerlessness and vulnerability increase.

- The survivor can make no sense of the loss. There is a great need to find meaning and attach blame.

- There is no opportunity for closure in the relationship.

- The symptoms of grief and shock are more intense than in normal grief and persist for a longer time.

- The trauma of the death can elicit Post Traumatic Stress Disorder (PTSD).

When the nurse-healer is aware of the issues involved in traumatic death, a more accurate assessment of the mourner is possible. Interventions can then be planned that facilitate, rather than hinder, healing.

Post Traumatic Stress Disorder

The client must be assessed carefully to detect if the symptoms of PTSD are present. In all losses, a form of psyche numbing occurs. In traumatic death, these feelings intensify. The survivor of traumatic death feels helpless and powerless. These feelings of helplessness and powerlessness may progress to PTSD (Rando, 1994).

Some individuals, however, when faced with the most traumatic circumstances, do not develop PTSD. These individuals move through the grief experience without suffering the intense emotions manifested in PTSD.

Nurses must be aware of the possibility of PTSD and be alert for the presence of symptoms. Recurrent, terror-filled nightmares, psychological distress, sleep disturbances, or chronic anxiety should alert the nurse to the possibility of PTSD. Failure to identify these symptoms can further complicate the healing process, because until the symptoms of PTSD are dealt with, grief lingers and cannot be resolved (Rando, 1994).

Nurses must help the survivor to deal with the effects of the trauma before the survivor can effectively work through the grief of the loss of the loved one. Successfully laying aside the traumatic experience requires help from several sources. The griever experiencing symptoms of PTSD needs to be evaluated by a psychiatrist or psychiatric clinical nurse specialist. The nurse can work closely with the client and other mental health professionals to facilitate healing.

Communication techniques are paramount along with a trusting nurse-client relationship. Without a therapeutic nurse-client relationship, the survivor will not trust the nurse enough to allow the truth to emerge. Support groups with those experiencing similar life circumstances can provide a healing atmosphere where survivors can work through their feelings.

The treatment goal in PTSD is to assist the griever to bring into conscious awareness the traumatic incident until the mind is dulled to the consequences of the event. Most often, the traumatic event must be dealt with first, then grieving can go on. At other times, dealing with the trauma and the grief can occur simultaneously (Rando, 1993).

All individuals working through grief must express and work through every intense emotion. PTSD is no exception. The terror, horror, anger, guilt, and helplessness must be fully ventilated and examined. The griever must learn to deal with anger constructively. New coping mechanisms must be learned or old coping mechanisms reactivated. The griever must be guided to create meaning out of the incident. Inappropriate assumptions of self-blame and guilt must be relinquished. Survivors must again establish meaningful and caring relationships with others (Rando, 1993).

Relationships Following Traumatic Death

Detachment can occur in families who lose loved ones from sudden unexpected death. Detachment means "a process whereby people withdraw and feel emotionally distant from each other" (Reed, 1993, p. 206). Initially, the survivors after a tragic death feel supportive of each other. During the first stages of bereavement before the funeral and immediately after the funeral, a close comforting environment often exists. However, as time passes, detachment can occur.

This detachment occurs more commonly in survivors who experience close ties within the family unit before death (Reed, 1993). The unexpected nature of death and the emotions generated by death produce a numbing effect. This numbing results in the survivors building protective cocoons by withdrawing from family members. Families cease to talk since to do so increases the pain of loss.

The role played by the victim within the family unit is void, leaving an emptiness in the family relationships that existed before the death. Rather than adapt to the changes in relationships within the family and support each other, family members withdraw. Those suffering the most intense grief experience more detachment from family.

Family support plays a significant role, particularly if the support is continued after the initial phase of grief. Time spent together discussing feelings allows the family unit to remain intact. Without family support, those suffering from intense grief feel even more detached. Lack of support from family members can result in hostility and anger directed at family members and increasing detachment (Lukas & Seiden, 1987).

Nurse-healers can intervene by providing safe avenues in which survivors can ventilate feelings that cannot be expressed within the family unit. Through active listening and supportive guidance, the nurse can minimize withdrawal from the family. With time, individual family members will begin to openly express their grief, first to the nurse, then to the other family members. Family counseling or support groups may facilitate this process.

SUMMARY

Any death, even anticipated death, is a traumatic experience to the surviving loved ones. Unanticipated death, such as a death from a heart attack, aneurysm, or stroke, leaves survivors shocked and bereaved. Most often, the grievers are capable of working through the grieving process without complications.

Complicated grief is associated with traumatic death such as death caused by homicide, suicide, or an accident. While traumatic death does not necessarily predispose the survivor to complications in mourning, survivors suffer emotions of greater intensity than those associated with normal grief.

When loved ones die violently, the grievers may suffer from traumatic imagery. Traumatic imagery is reliving the terror of the incident or imagining the feelings of horror felt by the victim. Traumatic imagery is a common occurrence with traumatic death. Such thoughts, coupled with intense grief, can lead to PTSD. Unless this problem is recognized and the survivors encouraged to express the intense feelings, they will not be able to progress through a more normal grieving process.

The loss of a loved one to suicide is frequently compounded by feelings of blame by the survivors. They feel guilty for failing to recognize clues that may have enabled them to help the victim. These feelings may turn to anger at the victim for failing to hold on or for inflicting unnecessary pain on loved ones. Shame at having a suicide in the family may be present.

In other instances where others are perceived to be directly or indirectly responsible for the death, survivors may experience additional feelings of anger and blame. These feelings may be directed toward those perceived to have caused the death. Some survivors have a strong need to assign blame. If someone or something else can be blamed, then the survivors can rid themselves of any responsibility.

Nurses play an important role in assisting the mourners in developing an understanding of the normal grieving process and the complex feelings exhibited when grief becomes more complicated. Nurses with a good understanding of both normal grief and complicated grief will be better prepared to assist the survivors than nurses who believe that all grief is the same.

REFLECTIONS

1. Think of a traumatic death recently publicized in the media. What feelings would you have if someone you loved were a victim of this trauma?

2. How would you talk to a family who had lost a mother or father through suicide? Have you ever contemplated suicide?

3. What methods of support do you feel would be most appropriate if a client you were working with expresses symptoms of PTSD?

4. What types of traumatic death do you fear the most?

References

American Psychiatric Association. (1994). *Diagnostic and Statistical Manual of Mental Disorders* (4th ed.). Washington, DC: Author.

Calhoun, L., Selby, J., & Selby, L. (1982). The psychological aftermath of suicide: An analysis of current evidence. *Clinical Psychology Review, 2,* 409–420.

Dunn, R., & Morrish-Vidners, D. (1987–88). The psychological and social experience of suicide survivors. *Omega, 18*(3), 175–213.

Faberow, N., Gallagher-Thompson, D., Gilewski, M., & Thompson, L. (1992). The role of social support in the bereavement process of surviving spouses of suicide and natural death. *Suicide and Life-Threatening Behavior, 22,* 107–121.

Figley, C. (1985). Introduction. In C. Figley (Ed.), *Trauma and its wake: The study and treatment of post-traumatic stress disorder.* New York: Brunner/Mazel.

Harowitz, M., Bonanno, G., & Hollen, A. (1993). Pathological grief: Diagnosis and explanation. *Psychosomatic Medicine, 55,* 260–273.

Lightner, C., & Hathaway, N. (1990). *Giving sorrow words*. New York: Warner Books, Inc.

Lukas, C., & Seiden, H. M. (1987). *Silent grief: Living in the wake of suicide*. New York: Charles Scribner's Sons.

O'Hara, C. (1970). *Fundamentals of criminal investigation*. Springfield, IL: Charles C. Thomas.

Rando, T. (1993). *Treatment of complicated mourning*. Champaign, IL: Research Press.

Rando, T. (1994). Complications in mourning traumatic death. In I. B. Corless, B. B. Germino, & M. Pittman (Eds.), *Dying, death, and bereavement* (pp. 253–271). Boston: Jones and Bartlett Publishers.

Reed, M. (1993). Suicide and life threatening behavior. *The American Association of Suicidology, 23*(3), 204–222.

Rynearson, E., & McCleery, J. (1993). Bereavement after homicide: A synergism of trauma and loss. *American Journal of Psychiatry, 150*(2), 258–261.

Wolfelt, A. (1991, March/April). Toward an understanding of complicated grief: A comprehensive overview. *The Journal of Hospice and Palliative Care*, 28–30.

Welue, T. (1975). Preventing pathological bereavement. In B. Schoenbert, I. Gerber, A. Wiener, A. Kutscher, D. Peretz, & A. Carr (Eds.), *Bereavement: Its psychological aspects*. New York: Columbia Press.

8 CHRONIC SORROW: CARING FOR LOVED ONES WITH A CHRONIC ILLNESS OR DISABILITY

Beatriz C. Nieto and Sally S. Roach

When sorrows come, they come not single . . .
but in battalions.

Hamlet IV v. 78

INTRODUCTION

In the previous chapters, we have defined loss, bereavement, grief, and mourning. We have looked at and described normal and abnormal reactions to grief, loss of a spouse, children and grief, and those who have suffered the loss of a loved one due to a traumatic event.

Common to each type of loss and bereavement discussed thus far is the finality of the situation. The inevitable becomes reality and the survivors are left to grieve the loss of a loved one.

It is evident that experiencing a loss is one of the most difficult tasks that all of us will experience. Dealing with death and dying is a journey filled with heartache, disappointment, guilt, anger, and frustration, at times laced with the hope of what we wish would be instead of how things really are.

This chapter focuses on chronic sorrow. Chronic sorrow is the term used to express a never-ending sorrow, a sorrow characterized by no predictable end and no true resolution. This type of sorrow is filled with peaks and valleys. Chronic sorrow has been described as a prolonged feeling of loss and bereavement that can be attributed to a chronic illness or disease. Reed and Leonard (1989) described the attributes of chronic sorrow as episodic pain and sadness that is (a) variable in intensity at different times for a person and also between persons and situations; (b) permanent, recurs for the lifetime of the disabled person; and (c) interwoven with periods of neutrality, satisfaction, and happiness.

The concept of chronic sorrow was first used to identify the heartache experienced in the lives of parents with a disabled child (Olshansky, 1962). The grief these parents feel, rather than following a predictable pattern of ups and downs leading to adjustment and acceptance, becomes a continual campaign to deal with the tremendous responsibilities and stresses involved in caring for a disabled child. Their lives are characterized by peaks and valleys as the child progresses at her own pace and not as other children. Each milestone may bring back the grief of the loss of that perfect child the parents envisioned before the birth. A deep sadness and pain may occur when the efforts of a disabled child to meet a milestone or developmental task never quite reach the mastery of other children. While there is joy in the accomplishments of a disabled child, there is an underlying sorrow that lingers and causes pain and sadness.

Chronic sorrow is not limited to parents caring for a disabled child. It also includes the sorrow experienced by the families of a person who has a chronic disease, such as the sorrow and grief of a man watching his wife progress through the downward spiral of Alzheimer's disease or the wife of a man diagnosed with multiple sclerosis. Any chronic disease or disability that is long lasting and pervasive in the lives of the family members can provide the roots of chronic sorrow.

Chronic sorrow or periodic recurrence of sadness is a common response when loss of a relationship of attachment is due to a permanent disability that renders the individual forever changed from the hoped-for child or from the known person (Worthington, 1989). Fraley (1986) suggested that chronic sorrow is a part of the normal grief response that follows an event of life-long implications for the caregiver.

ESSENTIAL COMPONENTS OF CHRONIC SORROW

Essential components of chronic sorrow help to define the boundaries and provide insight for caregivers working with families in situations where chronic sorrow is likely to occur. With chronic sorrow, the losses are continually redefined in new situations with new problems and trigger feelings of sadness and grief (Lindergren, Burke, Hainsworth, & Eakes, 1992). Essential components of chronic sorrow as identified by Teel (1991) include:

- The loss results from an occurrence other than death.

- There is a negative contrast between the past idealized state and the present actual state.

- No positive change in the situation is recognized as a future possibility.

- Certain trigger events clearly identify the disparity between the past idealized state and the present or the actual state.

Chronic sorrow has also been described as being timeless, with a cyclic and progressive nature.

Chronic Sorrow Is Timeless

The timelessness of chronic sorrow comes more clearly into focus when parents with a severely disabled child must think and plan beyond their own deaths to see that the child is cared for and, hopefully, loved. Although many disabled children do not outlive their parents, the thought of who will care for the child or what will happen to the child if the parents should die first becomes another source of worry for those in the midst of chronic sorrow.

Chronic Sorrow Is Cyclic

The cyclic nature of chronic sorrow can be seen each time a disabled child fails to reach a developmental milestone. Some of the major milestones the child is unable to accomplish often include the ability to talk at the expected time, to walk, to crawl, to start school, or to learn to read. The unkind remarks and the stares of both other children and thoughtless adults add to the grief experienced by the parents. Wiker, Wasow, and Hatfield (1981) studied the concept of chronic sorrow by exploring the grief experienced by parents of retarded children. The study found the grief patterns of parents were a series of ups and downs. Parents depicted the later stages of development as even more painful than the early years of the child's life.

Chronic Sorrow Is Progressive

The progressive nature of chronic sorrow was brought into question by Martinson (as cited in Lindgre, Burke, Hainsworth, & Eakes, 1992). Although chronic sorrow may progress in intensity in some instances, many people suffering from chronic sorrow live more in a relative constant state of sadness, characterized by highs and lows. The intensity does not necessarily increase, but its omnipotent nature pervades every aspect of life.

Sharon's Story

Sharon's first emotion when learning of her pregnancy was joy. How wonderful it would be to have a tiny baby! But her joy quickly turned to unspeakable sadness when Teri was born. She could not believe it. How could she and John have such a child? Sharon found herself not wanting to hold Teri or even touch him. That instant bond so often discussed was not there. She felt so guilty and so sad. Here was a tiny creature who was not lovable, and yet who needed love so desperately.

With time, although her sadness had not dissipated, Sharon began to bond with Teri. She looked forward to seeing him, to touching him, and to giving him love. Adjustment was not easy. At times, the incredible feeling of sadness would overtake Sharon and she would weep uncontrollably. Sharon realized how demanding it was to care for a child with special needs. Both Sharon and John found that they had to totally restructure their lives, their goals for their child, and their own goals. Sharon had always thought that she would go back to graduate school, but now that seemed out of the question.

Being with other parents and children near Teri's age is sometimes difficult for Sharon. She sees the other children walking, talking, and running. She knows that Teri will never be able to do these things or if he can, his physical disabilities will limit his skills to those of a child much younger than he. Sharon's life is a series of ups and downs, highs and lows. She finds herself thinking of the day Teri first held his cup and drank from it. Sharon was so happy for him and he was so proud of himself, but her joy was short-lived when she saw a child much younger than Teri do the same thing. Sometimes she asks, "Why me? Why Teri? Doesn't he deserve better? Doesn't he deserve to be simply normal?" Sharon feels intense pain and fear at the thought of something happening to her or John. "Who would love him as we do, care for him as we do, rejoice at his accomplishments?" "What would happen to him if we were not here?" There is truly no end to the pain.

CHRONIC ILLNESS

Chronic sorrow is not limited to the sorrow experienced by parents of disabled children; it is also experienced by those who suffer from chronic illness or long-term disability. Chronic illness is the irreversible presence, accumulation, or latency of disease states or impairments that involve the total human environment for supportive care and self-care, maintenance of function, and prevention of further disability (Lubkin, 1990, p. 6). Chronic illness occurs at all ages and stages of development. From infancy to old age, chronic illness affects the lives of all involved.

Chronic illness has been characterized as being the number one health problem in the United States. It is not uncommon to find people afflicted with one or more chronic conditions

(Forsyth, Delancy, & Gresham, 1984). The type and severity of the chronic illness determines the amount of physical and/or mental limitation that may be experienced. In some, the chronic condition may limit the ability to perform certain activities of daily living. In others, the chronic condition may be serious enough to prevent the person from carrying out major activities like attending school or holding down a job (Reif & Estes, 1982).

Chronic illness can take many different forms. For example, chronic illness may occur suddenly or through an insidious process. It can have episodic flare-ups, exacerbations, or remain in remission (Lubkin, 1990). In order to illustrate the impact chronic illness has on those afflicted and those involved in their care, several examples follow.

Infancy to Adolescence

Chronic illness afflicts persons in all age groups, including children. A child may suffer from congenital defects, sensory impairments, mental retardation, learning behavior disorders, as well as disorders affecting the respiratory system. The latter are often considered the most common type of disorders afflicting children. Any of these disorders, depending upon their prevalence and severity, will have a tremendous impact upon the child's physical as well as mental growth and development.

Colm O'Brien

The day Colm O'Brien was born was the happiest day for his parents and grandparents, for Colm was the first male child born into the family. He was a happy baby, healthy in all respects, until he was about 14 months old. At that age, he began experiencing repeated upper respiratory infections which required frequent visits to the pediatrician. "Bronchitis," the doctor would say. "It should clear up with this antibiotic." It would clear up, but only a few weeks later he would develop a cough, congestion, and be off to the doctor once more. It soon developed into a vicious cycle that never seemed to end.

Colm's condition got progressively worse, requiring nebulizer treatments and frequent trips to the emergency room. When he was 3 years old, his pediatrician referred the family to an allergist who specialized in treating children with asthma and allergies. Colm was diagnosed with asthma and the family was also told he was allergic to several things. After that diagnosis, there were weekly allergy shots, daily medications, and the continued dread that Colm would suffer a major setback, which often resulted in hospitalization for several days.

Being in the hospital was hard for Colm as well as his family. His parents took turns staying at the hospital with him. It devastated them to see Colm struggling with every breath. His mom would question in her mind why it had to be her son. She found herself making bargains with God if only her son could be free from this asthma. After a few days, usually 3 to 4, Colm would be released from the hospital. Once at home, the strict regimen of treatments, medications, and weekly allergy shots began again. Colm's parents learned to administer prescribed treatments (e.g., nebulizer, air purifier, humidifier, vaporizer), bought all the necessary equipment, and were willing to try almost anything, to the point of being obsessed with trying to prevent Colm from suffering another acute episode of asthma.

It has been 7 years since Colm was diagnosed as having asthma. He will be 11 years old soon. It has not been easy for Colm and his family. At the first sign of coughing, congestion, or throat irritation, his mom is still quick to take him to the doctor for a checkup. She often feels that she is overprotective, but she does not like to take any chances. She feels frustrated and helpless when Colm's health takes a turn for the worse. She gets a pain at the pit of her stomach when she hears him wheezing and having trouble breathing. She sometimes feels like she is drowning and can't catch her breath.

Colm is also tired of having to take medications, treatments, and allergy shots. He often asks his mom why he has to be sick all the time, why he has to take so many medications, and why he can't be like other kids. How can such questions be answered? In spite of his many bouts with asthma, frequent infections, and rigid medication regimen, Colm is a bright, energetic child who enjoys camping out, playing basketball, hanging out with his friends, and playing the piano. He has learned to deal with his illness through the years. His family has learned to care for him and to cope with the illness by not focusing only on the negative aspects. Colm and his family take one day at a time and are grateful for every day that he feels well and remains healthy.

When a child suffers from a chronic illness, maintaining the prescribed medical regimen often becomes the major focus of the parents as well as the child. The time required to maintain a medical regimen may conflict with a child's growth and developmental needs. In infancy, for example, the amount of time parents spend interacting with their child will influence the infant's mental as well as physical growth and development. It is during infancy that a relationship of trust and security is established between parent and child. Often the early establishment of trust and security is interrupted due to separations that may occur because of frequent hospitalizations, testing, and/or necessary treatments.

As the child grows older, her focus expands outward and she begins to seek interactions with peers and other adults besides her parents. It is during the preschool and school-age years that a child's self-awareness and self-value begin to develop. Maintaining a normal lifestyle may be difficult because of the interference of treatment procedures and scheduling of medical regimen.

When an adolescent suffers from a chronic illness, he faces the dual role of normal adult development and acceptance of a life with limitations (Lubkin, 1990). There are certain problem areas that a young person afflicted with a chronic illness will be faced with throughout his lifetime. Dunlop (1982) identified the following problem areas:

- the uncertainty of the future

- identification with the illness and the sick role

- taking negative risks

- illness and death as unexpected life events

- dependence/independence conflicts with parents

- being different

The chronic condition of asthma and allergies presented in the vignette about Colm illustrates only one of many diseases that afflict children. It is important to remember that chronic illness not only affects the child's life but has an impact on the lives of every family member. The survival of children into young adulthood can be attributed to devoted family members, cooperation with complicated therapeutic regimens, and advances in medical technology (Lubkin, 1990).

Young to Middle-Aged Adults

The young to middle-aged adult years are characterized as being the most productive time in a person's life. It is during this time that individuals are launching careers and marriages, beginning and raising families, experiencing changes in status, and preparing for retirement (Lubkin, 1990).

Common illnesses that afflict adults include arthritis, hypertension, diabetes, heart conditions, and respiratory diseases. When a family member is afflicted with a chronic illness, the whole family will suffer or share in the experience. Energy that should be spent on careers, marriage, and family may have to be used to cope with the illness and its many demands. The illness may interfere with the conception and completion of long-term plans, goals, and dreams. The following vignette depicts the impact chronic illness can have during this stage of growth and development.

Manuel Maria Mendez

Manuel Maria Mendez was diagnosed with diabetes when he was 32 years old. The diagnosis was a great devastation to him because he had never really been ill before. He had no idea what impact this disease would have on his health, family, and life.

Manuel was diagnosed when he went for his annual physical. His fasting blood sugar was over 350. After obtaining the results, the physician called Manuel and told him that he needed to be hospitalized at once in order to run further tests to confirm the diagnosis and begin to regulate his blood sugar levels. During the hospitalization Manuel began to get a glimpse of changes that he would have to undergo in order to control his diabetes. The severity of the diagnosis became more apparent to him as the nurses, dietician, and doctors came in to talk to him about diabetes, insulin injections, diet, exercise, and so many other things. They talked to him about control, not cure. They told him he should be able to live a healthy, normal life. For the first time in his life, Manuel was fearful of the future. Was his future to be filled with frequent ailments, insulin injections, and hospitalizations? What about his family, his children, and his plans for the future? Many thoughts swirled through his mind.

Gradually, after several years of living with diabetes, Manuel and his family have learned to take one day at a time and live life to its fullest. Although his days are filled with making diet plans, monitoring his blood sugar, and giving himself insulin injections, as well as frustrations, fear, and sometimes anger, Manuel has learned what is really important in his life. His priorities have changed. He no longer takes his life or his family for granted. He has learned that maintaining adequate control of his diabetes allows him to establish a balance between life, family, and work.

Older Adults

Older adults are the population most often affected by chronic illness. Individuals in this age group are usually diagnosed with several chronic health problems. According to Soldo and Manton (1985), common chronic conditions of persons over age 65 include arthritis, hypertensive disease, hearing impairments, heart conditions, chronic sinusitis, visual impairments, arteriosclerosis, diabetes mellitus, and varicose veins. It is estimated that approximately 2 million elderly people need assistance with one or more activities of daily living and about 5 million people are involved in caring for elderly family members (Brody, 1985).

The following vignette depicts the sorrow expressed by a nurse as her mother-in-law's physical and mental capacities diminished with Alzheimer's disease.

The Cloak of Grief

When I first heard the diagnosis of Alzheimer's, I didn't even know what it was. As the doctor explained the basic idea of the expected deterioration and eventual death, I knew that as a nurse and the only female in the family, I would have to be the strong one. Now I understood why God led me through 19 years of experience with patients. I was thankful that I could do this for my precious mother-in-law. I thanked God for preparing me for the most important task of my life.

Though I was unaware, grief came into my life like a cloak to ward off a chill. The hood of the cloak was not needed initially. However, as the years wore on and my emotions became cooler, the cloak seemed to become a yoke that constantly weighed upon my shoulders.

As my mother-in-law deteriorated, more facets of her life became my responsibility. At times, I felt as though I was facing a one-way road toward my mother-in-law's death. I could not even turn right or left. The hood of the cloak seemed to somehow creep upon my head and cut off my peripheral vision. As I pulled the cloak closer around me, my hands were withdrawn to the inside of the cloak, only allowed out to give the necessary enemas, baths, and feedings, or to diaper and catheterize her. Friends, work, and family activities all seemed to drift to the side, allowing the hood to protect me from seeing the areas of my life I was neglecting. I thought God was allowing her to survive until I learned more patience. I tried to be less resentful of the time I missed with family and friends, particularly with my son, but exhaustion overtook me and I felt guilty and resentful.

Each step of her deterioration was followed by a time of grief. The steps turned into milestones when I felt the closeness, then the heaviness, and finally the constriction of that cloak. I particularly remember the day she could no longer remember my name. I came home to find her with two dresses on and with her bra over the second one. My bachelor brother-in-law had been too shy to change her. After I walked her to the bedroom and straightened her appearance, she marched back to the dining room and said, "That woman thinks I do not know anything about clothes." From that day forward, I was called "that woman."

With the slow, but persistent mental and physical deterioration of my mother-in-law, the cloak and hood seemed like a yoke that kept me at the door of ongoing and constant grief. It seemed I was living on the edge from one crisis to another. This ongoing grief was at my doorstep for over 13 years.

TIME-BOUND VS. CHRONIC SORROW

Two approaches to the reactions of parents and close family members to the crisis of adapting to a loved one with a disability or chronic illness have been identified. The first approach is the time-bound model proposed by Fortier and Wanlass in 1984. This model proposed five stages that parents go through in adjusting to the presence of a disabled child. The stages include impact, denial, grief, focusing attention, and closure. *Impact* is the initial stage and is manifested by fear and anxiety. The family is not prepared for this type of crisis and can become disjointed and disorganized. *Denial* is reached very quickly and serves as a buffer until the family can face the reality of the situation. As denial fades and reality drifts in, the family enters the third stage, that of *grief.* Grief can be exhibited in a variety of ways such as through anger, blame, sadness, or depression. When the family begins to develop coping skills, the next stage of *focusing outward* begins. In this stage, the family actively adapts to the illness or disability of the family member and the stage is set for *closure*. During closure, the family accepts the situation and incorporates coping mechanisms to effectively deal with the chronicity of the situation. The time-bound model proposes that the situation is a crisis that can be resolved by identifying coping mechanisms that lessen the impact of the crisis and enable adaptation.

Chronic sorrow, as proposed by Olshansky (1962), focuses on the process of adapting to the presence of a disabled child. For Olshansky, there is no real closure or ending to the emotional response experienced by parents of disabled children. The pain and grief are normal and natural responses. They will ebb and flow over a lifetime even though love, support, and care of the child may flourish. In effect, the parents never truly pass the impact stage. Guilt and anger may always be an underlying presence.

As was mentioned earlier, chronic sorrow is not limited to families of children with disabilities, but is a phenomenon present in situations in which loved ones have any number of chronic illnesses, such as multiple sclerosis, Alzheimer's disease, diabetes, or afflictions of a traumatic nature such as spinal cord injury or traumatic brain injury. Feelings of grief and pain vary in intensity for each family member involved. In situations where families are confronted daily with the source of the grief and no visible end to the situation, the natural response is that of chronic sorrow. They have before them each day a constant reminder of the source of their grief and they episodically experience and reexperience the pain and anguish of the grieving process. In order for adaptation to begin, the family must develop adequate coping strategies that allow some normalcy in life to continue. However, even with adaptation, periods of joy and happiness are marred by an underlying sadness that is ever present and ready to surface at a moment's notice.

THE ROLE OF THE NURSE-HEALER

Nurses in all work situations can take an active role in guiding, teaching, and supporting those who are experiencing chronic sorrow. Because nurses are in a unique position to work with the patient and family unit on a one-to-one basis, nurses can be instrumental in helping those who are faced with coping with chronic sorrow. Whether it be the wife of an elderly man with Alzheimer's disease, the mother of a pediatric patient with cerebral palsy, or a patient who has been diagnosed with cancer, diabetes, asthma, or a cardiac condition, nurses can use their skills as healers to guide the patient and her family to discover and recognize new health behaviors, make choices, and develop insight into how to cope effectively. In so doing, the nurse-healer assists the patient and the family to explore the purpose and find meaning in life. In finding purpose and meaning in the present moment, a patient's fullest potential can be realized (Dossey, 1988).

The nurse-healer can help bring to light the concerns and fears a patient and his family may be experiencing that are so often concealed. Nurses must be aware of the potential grief in every patient and/or family under their care. They must seek opportunities to draw both the patient and family members out to allow the expression of feelings. This catharsis will help the patient and his family be in congruence with inner resources, decrease stress, and enhance self-direction toward balance and harmony (Dossey, 1988).

The focus of care in chronic sorrow is on the family since chronic sorrow affects every member of the family to one degree or another. The ultimate goal is to make chronic sorrow manageable by teaching the family and the patient positive coping mechanisms in order to provide the highest possible functioning of the holistic being in the physical, mental, emotional, and spiritual aspects of life. With positive coping, the aspects of the disease or disability can be interwoven into all areas of everyday life, allowing adaptation to occur. Adjustment is a lifelong process that requires constant readjustment and enormous effort by each family member to keep some type of balance in the family unit.

Sensitivity of the nurse and other members of the health care team is of utmost importance. As one mother explained, "When Sue (the nurse) walked into the room her very presence gave me comfort. We had hardly talked at all when I felt that I could trust her. I do not even remember the words she spoke. I just knew that this was someone who cared about me and my baby." Sensitivity is a quality to be sought by the nurse and can be developed through sensitivity training and increased knowledge of the aspects of chronic sorrow. As the sensitivity of the nurse increases so will the ability of the nurse to model and transfer that sensitivity to other members of the health care team as well as the patient's family members.

STRATEGIES TO ENHANCE COPING

Positive coping strategies are essential if adaptation is to occur. The nurse evaluates past and present coping skills of the family and offers suggestions to enhance coping. The nurse and family collaborate to identify strengths and weaknesses and determine additional coping strategies. Strategies that can enhance coping include providing information, teaching self-care, providing emotional support, setting goals, and finding meaning in illness (Smeltzer & Bare, 1992).

Providing Information

Providing the patient and the family with accurate information and education on the disorder and characteristics of chronic sorrow can help to relieve anxiety and uncertainty as well as increase the sense of control of the individual in any given situation. Knowledge provides the patient and the family with the foundation to make honest and meaningful decisions concerning care, enables the family to identify feelings as natural and acceptable, and paves the way for the development of additional coping mechanisms. Encouragement can be gained from talking with others in similar situations. Learning the coping methods others use to survive can be useful in the process of adaptation.

Knowledge of the general time frames when certain reactions can be anticipated helps decrease feelings of helplessness. For example, when parents realize that it is normal for grief and anguish to resurface as the disabled child passes through important developmental milestones, they are better prepared to deal with these feelings when they occur.

The nurse must provide an atmosphere in which the patient and family feel comfortable asking questions and discussing feelings. Dialogue is encouraged and opportunities are provided for family members to ask questions.

Teaching Self-Care

Teaching self-care is a necessity when there is a disability involved. The more an individual is allowed to do and is able to do in caring for herself, the greater the self-esteem and sense of control. Most patients, no matter how severely disabled or ill, can meet some of their self-care needs. Needs that cannot be met by the patient can be met by the family. Allowing family members to participate in the care often relieves some of the anxiety and guilt.

Self-care takes a different focus for family members who are involved in the care. Often neglect of self becomes a difficulty. The caregiver gives so much of himself that all individuality is lost. Neglect of self represents a danger point for the caregiver and is a situation that requires intervention by the nurse-healer. The caregiver must be taught that self-care is an essential aspect of his own adjustment.

Providing Emotional Support

A beneficial coping skill for the patient is identifying the need for emotional support and having the courage to seek that support. Sometimes feelings of fear and detachment hinder families from seeking emotional support. The nurse-healer can begin to provide emotional support even before the patient identifies this as a need. The very presence of the nurse can sometimes contribute to the emotional well-being of the patient. Availability and willingness to listen are attributes necessary for dealing with those immersed in chronic sorrow.

Another avenue for providing emotional support is through support groups or dialogue groups. Talking to others who have faced similar life crises often provides comfort, offers the opportunity to explore alternate strategies, and meets needs not easily addressed with those who do not share in similar experiences.

Setting Realistic Goals

Goal setting is an important aspect in developing positive coping behaviors. The most important aspect in goal setting is identifying realistic, attainable goals. Both the family and the patient must participate in the development of these goals. Collaboration between the nurse and the family in setting goals increases the potential for successful goal setting. When goals are accomplished, the feelings of powerlessness and anxiety commonly associated with chronic sorrow decrease.

Finding Meaning

Families must be able to find meaning in the pain and anguish they are suffering. Some find meaning through spiritual avenues such as involvement in a church or synagogue. For others, participating in research studies or writing journals or poems are methods of exploring and expressing the meaning of the illness (Smeltzer & Bare, 1992). Each of these avenues should be explored with the patient.

While searching for meaning, values and beliefs are often clarified or changed. For example, the search for meaning may bring a deeper appreciation of the simple things in life, such as the beauty of a sunset or the sound of the ocean.

The strategies discussed thus far are by no means all inclusive. The use of these strategies will open doors for the nurse-

---

- Identify ways to deal with anger and depression without damaging family relations.

- Role-play difficult situations.

- Learn stress-reducing techniques.

- Recognize incongruence between expectations and reality.

- Explore feelings concerning role changes and role reversal.

- Explore ways to enhance self-esteem.

- Capitalize on strengths.

- Realistically identify abilities and limitations.

- Identify recreational activities.

- Take time for self.

TABLE 8.1 **Chronic Sorrow: Effective Coping Strategies**

healer to explore other alternatives for the patient who is suffering with chronic sorrow. Strategies must be individualized and planned in collaboration with the patient and the family. Refer to Table 8.1 for additional coping strategies that may be used to assist with adaptation.

Once adaptation has begun and the family is focusing on effective coping skills, they will be better able to put the illness or the disability in perspective. However, adjustment is a life-long process and will require continuous adaptation and readaptation as milestones are reached and assorted problems are encountered.

SUMMARY

The causes of chronic sorrow are many and varied. Individuals and/or families that are faced with a chronic condition or disability will be challenged to learn, cope, and find some meaning to life. It is not an easy journey. The way is filled with many hills and valleys. Nurses can help make the journey more tolerable by providing support, education, and guidance. They can help provide focus and explore attainable goals. This may promote adaptation and management of the chronic condition or disability and decrease stress, anxiety, and powerlessness.

REFLECTIONS

1. Have you or someone close to you experienced chronic sorrow? If so, what were the most significant problems faced?

2. In what ways would a nurse be most effective in working with patients experiencing chronic sorrow?

3. Are you better able to identify patients who are potential candidates for chronic sorrow?

4. How can you incorporate the principles discussed in this chapter into your practice?

References

Brody, E. M. (1985). Patient care as a normative stress. *Gerontologist*, *26*, 19–29.

Dossey, B. M. (1988). Nurse as healer: Toward the inward journey. In B. M. Dossey, L. Keegan, C. E. Guzzetta, & L. G. Kolkmeier, *Holistic nursing: A handbook for practice* (pp. 39–53). Gaithersburg, MD: Aspen Publishers, Inc.

Dunlop, J. (1982). Critical problems facing young adults with cancer. *Oncology Nursing Forum*, *9*(3), 33–38.

Forsyth, G. L., Delancy, K. D., & Gresham, M. L. (1984). Vying for a winning position: Management style of the chronically ill. *J. Nurse Health*, *7*, 181–188.

Fortier, L. M., & Wanlass, R. L. (1984). Family crises following the diagnosis of a handicapped child. *Family Relations*, *33*, 13–24.

Fraley, A. M. (1986). Chronic sorrow in parents of premature children. *Children's Health Care*, *15*, 114–118.

Lindergren, C., Burke, M., Hainsworth, M., & Eakes, G. (1992). Chronic sorrow: A lifetime concept. *Scholarly Inquiry for Nursing Practice: An International Journal*, *6*(1), 27–42.

Lubkin, I. M. (1990). *Chronic illness: Impact and interventions.* Boston: Jones and Bartlett Publishers Inc.

Olshansky, S. (1962). Chronic sorrow: A response to having a mentally defective child. *Social Casework*, *43*, 190–193.

Reed, P. G., & Leonard, V. E. (1989). An analysis of the concept of self-neglect. *Advances in Nursing Science*, *12*(1), 39–53.

Reif, L., & Estes, C. L. (1982). Long-term care: New opportunities for professional nursing. In C. H. Aiken (Ed.), *Nursing in the 1980s: Crisis, opportunities, challenges* (pp. 147–181). Philadelphia: Lippincott.

Smeltzer, S., & Bare, B. (1992). *Brunner and Suddarth's Textbook of Medical Surgical Nursing* (7th ed.) (pp. 141–144). Philadelphia: Lippincott.

Soldo, B. J., & Manton, K. G. (1985). Health status and service needs of the oldest old: Current patterns and future trends. *Memor Fund Q/Health Soc*, *63*(2), 286–319.

Teel, C. (1991). Chronic sorrow: Analysis of the concept. *Journal of Advanced Nursing*, *16*, 1311–1319.

Wiker, L. M., Wasow, M., & Hatfield, Z. (1981). Chronic sorrow revisited: Parent vs. professional depiction of the adjustment of parents of mentally retarded children. *American Journal of Orthopsychiatry*, *51*(1), 63–70.

Worthington, R. C. (1989). The chronically ill child and recurring family grief. *The Journal of Family Practice, 29*(4), 397–400.

BEREAVEMENT CARE: A ROLE FOR NURSE-HEALERS

Sally S. Roach

Too often we underestimate the power of a touch, a smile, a kind word, a listening ear, an honest compliment, or the smallest act of caring, all of which have the potential to turn a life around.

Leo Buscaglia

INTRODUCTION

The initial chapters of this book explore the various theories of grief. Subsequent chapters cover different aspects of grief and expand knowledge in specific areas of grief. This chapter focuses on the nurse's role in bereavement care and the strategies for healing that can be used to assist the griever through the grieving process. If coping strategies are ineffective, grief may stagnate or maladaptive behavior may develop. In order to prevent maladaptive coping and to facilitate the grieving process, it is imperative that those who have suffered loss have the opportunity to participate in bereavement care.

BEREAVEMENT CARE

The skills required to care for a grieving family may not be the technical skills that are so important in the acute care setting. Equipment such as a stethoscope, a syringe, or a cardiac monitor are not the most important aspects of bereavement care. Bereavement care rests on the ability of the nurse to use herself therapeutically. The therapeutic use of self by the nurse guides the griever toward a return to wholeness or harmony in body, mind, and spirit. The nurse who views herself as a participant in the healing process must develop the qualities of the nurse-healer.

ATTRIBUTES OF A NURSE-HEALER

A nurse-healer combines components of the art of nursing and the scientific principles involved in the technical aspects of nursing. Scientific principles form the basis for treatment regimens and nursing actions. These are combined with the art of using the self to guide and support the patient/family to incorporate self-healing strategies into their lifestyles.

Dossey, Keegan, Guzzetta, and Kolkmeier (1995) described the attributes of a nurse-healer. These attributes can be divided into two general areas: (1) attributes relating to the healing of self and (2) attributes relating to developing healing relationships with patients and families. Specific qualities of the nurse-healer are listed in table 9.1. To attain the qualities of the nurse-healer, the nurse first focuses on the healing of self.

Qualities of the nurse-healer are necessary to promote healing and to develop a meaningful relationship with the bereaved. These characteristics foster a healing environment. When personal needs are met, the nurse is better prepared to help patients in overcoming grief. The holistic care of self precedes the ability of the nurse to provide a healing environment for others.

DEVELOPING SELF-CARE

Self-care begins with self-analysis in each dimension of the human potentials (see chapter 3). Spiritual, mental, emotional,

Attributes relating to self-care include:

- Awareness that self-healing is a continual process

- Commitment to self-development and personal growth

- Openness to self-discovery

- Model of positive aspects of self-care

Attributes relating to the patient/family include:

- Awareness that the nurse's presence is equally as important as technical skills

- Respect and love for the patient/family as unique and special

- Encouragement to work on life's issues

- Guidance in the discovery of options

- Realization of coping skills

- Sharing insight without imposing personal values

- Nonjudgemental

- Listening actively

TABLE 9.1   *Attributes of a Nurse Healer*

From *Holistic Nursing: A Handbook for Practice* (2nd ed.) by B. M. Dossey, L. Keegan, C. Guzzetta, and L. G. Kolkmeier, 1995, Gaithersburg, MD: Aspen Publishers, Inc. Adapted by permission.

physical, and relationship potentials are explored by the nurse seeking to become a nurse-healer.

The potential for healing self is greater than many realize. However, self-healing requires time, commitment, and effort. Exploring thoughts and feelings leads to an understanding of one's personal philosophy of life. Identification of a personal philosophy of life allows priorities to be determined and the meaning of life to be clarified. When this is accomplished, the nurse has a foundation to guide others toward health and wholeness.

Spiritual

The spiritual aspect is that part of us that seeks guidance or comfort from a power greater than ourselves. Moberg (1979) defined spiritual well-being as "the affirmation of life in a relationship with God, self, community, and environment that nurtures and celebrates wholeness." Techniques to explore and develop spirituality include:

- prayer

- meditation

- reading the Bible or a book on spirituality

- writing one's own philosophy of life

Exploring the following questions will help the nurse-healer in a self-analysis of spirituality:

Is spirituality an important part of my life?

How important is my relationship with God?

Why am I here?

What is my purpose in life?

What is my relationship to the universe?

What can I do to increase my spirituality?

Developing the spiritual aspect of self provides a serenity and calmness that bring into focus every other aspect of life.

Emotional

Love, tenderness, passion, fear, anger, and jealousy are all normal emotions. Emotions, for most of us, are mixed blessings. Emotions play a role in the accomplishment of life's greatest triumphs and in life's most heartbreaking tragedies. For example, the emotion of love is the overriding force responsible for a young man walking over 100 miles through snow-covered mountains to save his wife and child from certain death. On the other hand, the emotions of hate and anger that spur a husband to brutally murder his wife and child are emotions involved in one of life's most horrifying tragedies.

Emotions may arise from external or internal sources and are the expressions of our innermost feelings. While emotions are uncontrollable, our reactions to these emotions are controllable.

Nurses must explore their feelings to learn to express emotions in a way that is not destructive to themselves or to others.

Powell (1969) identified ways to manage emotions rather than allowing emotions to manage you. His suggestions include:

- Be aware of emotions. Thoughtfully and carefully identify exactly what emotions are felt.

- Admit emotions. Do not deny any emotion, be it anger, jealousy, resentment, love, care, or concern. Accept emotions as a natural and normal part of life.

- Investigate emotions. Trace the origin of emotions and honestly examine feelings.

- Acknowledge emotions. Do not rationalize or place blame. Simply acknowledge feelings (e.g., I feel angry, I feel hurt, or I feel sad).

- Integrate emotions. Make a judgment. Perhaps the choice will be to drop the topic, begin the discussion again, or adopt a nonjudgmental attitude. Integration allows control over the expression of the emotion.

The nurse desiring to become a nurse-healer must explore the following questions concerning emotions:

Am I able to identify my emotions?

How do I deal with my emotions?

Am I always in control?

Can I openly discuss my emotions?

Am I open to what others say?

Do I jump to conclusions?

What situations cause my emotions to get out of control?

Do I respect the feelings of others?

Physical

Caring for themselves in the physical realm is often an area neglected by nurses. Physical care includes caring for the body through proper rest, finding time for recreation, exercising, and eating a nutritious diet. Self-analysis of the physical aspects of care can lead to changes in lifestyle and movement toward better physical health. The nurse must ask:

What aspects of my lifestyle are unhealthy?

Do I model a healthy lifestyle?

What can I do to improve my lifestyle?

How can I more effectively model a healthy lifestyle?

Mental

In preparing to be a nurse-healer, the nurse must become knowledgeable in the care and treatment of patients. Learning never ceases and new knowledge and new techniques are continually developing. An openness to new ideas and the development of new skills is vital. The following questions must be examined:

Am I knowledgeable?

Do I continually strive to increase my knowledge?

Am I satisfied with the status quo?

What am I doing to stimulate my mind?

Am I open to new ideas?

Relationships

The ability to form a therapeutic relationship is critical to becoming a nurse-healer. Without the trust and confidence of the patient, the nurse cannot have a positive impact. For self-analysis in this realm, the following questions are considered:

Do I maintain satisfying relationships with others?

Am I open and honest with others?

Must I have all of the control?

Am I able to accept the thoughts and feelings of others even though they are different from my own?

Am I judgmental?

Do I have a balance between work and leisure?

The holistic care of self prepares the nurse to provide a healing environment for others.

THE PROCESS OF CONNECTING

Connecting is a term used to describe a type of bonding between the nurse and the client or family. When caring for those suffering from grief, forming a connection is particularly important since the most important therapeutic tool the nurse has is himself. The characteristics of the nurse-healer facilitate the process of connecting.

Connecting is defined as "transpersonal experiences and feelings that lead to the sense of connection, attachment, or bonding between a nurse and a patient or family" (Clayton, Murray, Horner, & Greene, 1991). For nurses involved in caring for the bereaved, connecting can be the catalyst that allows the nurse to develop a therapeutic relationship.

A study on connecting by Clayton et al. (1991) identified four stages of connecting: presencing, attending, affiliating, and empowering. According to Clayton et al., *presencing* allows both the nurse and the client or family to come together and interact. The nurse who is sensitive to the needs of the family and is available or present to help meet the needs can develop a strong presence.

Attending is evidenced by caring behaviors and technical skills exhibited by the nurse. *Affiliating* occurs as the process continues and a type of bonding occurs. In this stage, an awareness of increased trust and self-disclosure of the nurse and the family becomes apparent. A feeling that the nurse has gone beyond what is expected strengthens the bond and fosters loyalty.

The last stage is that of *empowering*. In this stage, the client/family becomes less dependent on the nurse. As positive coping behaviors develop, the client or the family gains confidence to act independently and decisively (Clayton et al., 1991). Nurses who connect with those in their care are in a better position to develop more meaningful relationships.

DEVELOPING A HEALING RELATIONSHIP

Recovering from the death of a loved one is an extremely powerful and intense human experience. Few who have suffered the emotional turmoil of grief are left unchanged. Nurses can provide the support and guidance necessary to guide the griever through the grieving process. In order for a healing relationship to develop, the nurse and the client must form a bond or connection as discussed in the previous section. This healing relationship will aid the nurse in identifying and developing strategies necessary for the griever to recover from the loss. With a healing relationship, the nurse and the client feel free to explore options and formulate goals.

Assistance with the grieving process can be done in a formal or an informal setting. An informal setting may be the most practical since the relationship often began before the loss occurred. However, a structured setting may be most effective since the client can be followed more closely and progress can be evaluated more effectively.

Entry into a nurse-client relationship occurs with the first session. At the initial session, the nurse performs an assessment of the client's needs. Avenues to explore during the initial session include: the circumstances of the death, the relationship of the client with the deceased, any prior losses and coping mechanisms used, physical and psychological symptoms present, relationship with other family members, spiritual needs, and identification of those who can provide support.

At this first session, the nurse may also choose to discuss the normal aspects of grief and what the client can expect. Goals or outcomes are discussed and various healing strategies are presented for consideration. The client and the nurse mutually agree on the strategies to use. The client may be given an assignment to be completed before the next session. Assignments such as beginning a journal or reading a portion of a book or an article on grief may be helpful.

A schedule is developed in which the client is to be seen regularly. Subsequent sessions are based on the client's individual needs and where the client is in the grieving process. The nurse develops a plan of care based on the assessment gleaned from the initial interview. If needed, goals and strategies can be modified or changed to facilitate healing.

At each session, the nurse assesses diet, sleep patterns, and exercise. If a need in any of these areas is identified, the nurse discusses options and ways in which these needs can be more fully met.

A FRAMEWORK FOR HEALING

The healing process can be examined using any of the theories discussed in chapter 1. William Worden's theory was selected because his tasks for successful grieving provide a framework for the nurse to plan healing strategies and to evaluate progress. Worden (1982) identified four tasks mourners must accomplish for successful grieving. These tasks are:

- accept the reality of the loss
- experience the pain of the loss
- rediscover meaning in life without the loved one
- reinvest in life

If successful grieving is viewed as a series of tasks to accomplish, then grieving must be an active, not passive, process. An active process requires work and effort to succeed. Choices are made by the griever that will hinder or support the grieving process.

Attig (1991) viewed grief as a passive emotion and grieving as an active process. When grieving, the client is actively engaged in the work of developing healing strategies. Actively working through grief requires that the griever relinquish the overwhelming desire to bring the loved one back to life. When the griever relinquishes the loved one, she is ready to begin to work toward the development of healing strategies necessary to overcome grief (Attig, 1991). Worden's tasks can be used as a framework in working with the client as she actively progresses through the grieving process.

Accepting the Reality of the Loss

Accepting the reality of the loss can be extremely painful and for some quite lengthy. Denial is the initial response for almost everyone faced with the death of a loved one. Denial provides an avenue of escape until the bereaved can face the emotional pain that occurs with the death. Some will pass quickly through denial, while others will progress slowly, lingering over every detail of the death. Confusion, the inability to concentrate, and numbness characterize this stage of grief.

There is often a strong need to relate the details of death repeatedly. Repeating the incident may provide a pathway through which acceptance of the death finally penetrates to the innermost being of the client. Healing strategies used by the nurse-healer to help the client accept the reality of the loss include:

- actively listening to the client's comments

- using open-ended questions to encourage verbalization

- encouraging verbalization of the circumstances surrounding the loss

Assessing for any physical symptoms (chest pain, abdominal pain, fatigue, difficulty breathing, insomnia, and so on) and for psychological symptoms such as anxiety, depression, apathy, and anger is also important. The presence of these symptoms suggests problems with accepting the reality of the loss and they need to be addressed. When the reality of the death is accepted, the client is ready to go on to the next phase of the healing process.

Experiencing the Pain of the Loss

As the numbness and denial subside, the intense pain of the grieving process begins. This is where the real grief work identified by Lindemann (1944) begins. Remembering, reliving, and thinking about the deceased plays a major part in experiencing the pain. Suppression of the pain lengthens the process of grief and delays progress. Emotions commonly felt during grief include anger, depression, and guilt.

Learning to express anger is often difficult. When a loved one dies, anger is often masked by feelings of guilt or depression. Expression of anger is necessary for healing to begin. Anger can be directed toward the self for not doing enough to help the deceased, for not providing enough support, or for an imagined indiscretion. Anger can be directed at the deceased for dying or for not providing for the family after death. Family members, health care providers, or God may also be the focus of anger.

Vargas, Loya, and Hodde-Vargas (1989) theorized that when anger is generalized, the griever continues to struggle with his emotions. Unfocused anger causes grief to stagnate. However, as the anger becomes more focused toward the deceased, the griever is better able to accept the reality of the death. As the reality of death is accepted, the griever can move toward relinquishing the loved one. When anger becomes focused on the deceased, the griever can see the anger as illogical and inappropriate.

The release of anger acts as a cathartic to penetrate the barriers of grief. The griever must be assured that anger is normal and part of the healing process. Techniques to release anger and rage include role playing, hitting a pillow or a punching bag, crying, and speaking to an empty chair.

A form of Gestalt therapy, the empty chair is a method popularized by Frederick Perls (1951). In Gestalt therapy, the clients are helped to recognize feelings and emotions blocked from awareness and bring them into the open. At times, conflicts and life issues become the focus. The empty chair technique may be used with the grieving client to clarify emotions, release anger, or resolve conflict. Following is a brief overview of the empty chair technique and its use with the grieving client. For a more thorough description of this intervention, the reader is referred to the work of Perls.

Talking to an empty chair involves placing two chairs facing each other. The client sits in one chair facing the empty chair. The client is asked to envision the deceased sitting in the opposite chair and is instructed to say whatever she wishes to the deceased in the "empty" chair. Emotions such as anger or guilt can be expressed. The pain of the loss may be expressed as well. After time has been allowed for expression of thoughts and feelings, the client is asked to change chairs and become the deceased. The client is instructed to respond as she feels the deceased would respond. During the dialogue, the nurse may interject statements that rephrase what the client is saying or provide the client with open-ended questions to provoke expression (Perls, 1951).

Another healing strategy is to ask the griever to write letters to the deceased. When completed, these letters may be taken to the cemetery or another significant place. They may be read over the grave, torn into small pieces, and allowed to blow away with the wind, or they may be buried. These activities are symbolic of freedom from the painful emotions associated with the death.

Depression and guilt are closely akin to anger and are, if not in the extreme, a normal part of grief. Symptoms of depression may be present and function to slow the bereaved down, allowing time for reflection. Symptoms of depression that would fall within the normal realm include feelings of sadness, changes in appetite, difficulty sleeping, or episodic weeping. The depression associated with grief seldom reaches a major depressive episode that requires medication or psychiatric intervention. Symptoms of the bereaved that would suggest a major depressive episode include: excessive guilt, suicidal ideation, preoccupation with worthlessness, psychomotor retardation, marked functional impairment, and hallucinatory experiences (American Psychiatric Association, 1994). Any of these symptoms indicate the need for evaluation by a psychiatric clinical nurse specialist or psychiatrist. Physical complaints similar to those of the deceased, progressive social isolation, psychosomatic illness, substance abuse, or addictive behaviors also suggest the need for a more extensive evaluation.

Depression, anger, and guilt are common emotions of grief. The most effective method of working through emotional pain is verbalization, exploration, acceptance, and forgiveness of self and others. Healing strategies employed by the nurse include:

- encouraging verbalization of feelings and emotions

- providing avenues for the expression of anger, guilt, resentment, or pain

- validating the normalcy of emotions

- reviewing past coping mechanisms

- identifying maladaptive coping mechanisms

- forgiving self and others

- reviewing and remembering shared experiences

Reviewing and remembering shared experiences between the lost loved one and the griever provides the griever time to explore emotional needs met by the deceased. Adjusting to life without the loved one entails finding alternate ways to meet the emotional needs previously met by the deceased. Needs met by the deceased must be clarified before healing strategies can be effective.

Rediscovering Meaning in Life

The period of rediscovering meaning in life is filled with yearning, searching, and discovery. The griever yearns for the loved one to return so the old way of life can resume. The griever searches for ways to provide some type of normalcy to everyday life. Finally, the griever discovers meaning for the death. Yearning, searching, and discovering all play a significant role during this phase of grief. An exact meaning for why the death occurred may not be identified. For example, no meaning may ever be found concerning why the death of a child occurred. However, a new, different or modified meaning to the reason for the griever's existence or to life may be found.

During this period, socialization is encouraged. Friends, family, or support groups allow verbalization of feelings, validation of what is normal, and provide the opportunity to compare reactions and feelings. This interaction aids in the search for meaning.

If religion plays a significant role in the individual's life, encouragement is given to attend religious services and participate in religious activities. Individuals who participate in religious activities appear to have an increased ability to find meaning in life. These individuals also seem to adjust more easily to the loss of a loved one (McIntosh, Silver, & Wortman, 1993).

The meaning of any event to an individual is unique and personal. Every aspect of life has meaning regardless of the individual's ability to identify the meaning. The griever is encouraged to actively seek meaning because meaning makes life richer and fuller (Dossey et al., 1995).

In the grieving process when meaning is identified, the death makes sense. Giving meaning empowers the griever to develop the healing strategies that pave the way for reinvestment in life and resolution of the grief. However, for some the search for meaning for the actual death is elusive and no meaning is ever identified (Wortman & Silver, 1989). Some may never find acceptable answers to the questions: "Why did my child have to die?" "Why did God allow this to happen?" They may, however, find a new or different meaning in life.

Grief work during this stage is physically and emotionally exhausting (Curry & Stone, 1992). Symptoms such as fatigue, weight loss, weight gain, insomnia, or anxiety may develop. Depressive symptoms such as sadness, loss of interest in activities, or feelings of worthlessness may occur. Careful assessment by the nurse can lead to intervention before these symptoms become severe.

Crying is an avenue for the release of these emotions. A sensitive nurse sees the benefit of tears and is patient and accepting during these periods of emotional heartache.

Areas in which the nurse-healer may focus discussion are: life review, verbalization of experiences using photographs and sentimental keepsakes, reengaging in activities shared with the loved one, returning to special places shared with the deceased, attending special events, dealing with holidays, or identifying positive aspects of the future.

Reinvesting in Life

Reinvesting in life is closely akin to hope. Hope means confident expectation. The confident expectation, or hope, that the future can be full and happy, even without the deceased, is the goal for the griever at this stage. With confidence that the future can be good, the griever can let go of the emotional ties with the past and the fear of the future.

Letting go does not mean forgetting, but it will make remembrances of the past sweeter and more cherished. Memories bring a smile, not a tear; happiness, not sadness. With reinvestment in life, the griever is free to remember the good times shared, the lessons learned, and the love that will endure throughout life.

Social support is encouraged during all aspects of the grieving process. The role of social relationships peaks as the griever relinquishes the loved one that they have so tenaciously held onto and reaches out to others to reinvest in life. Suggestions to help the griever reinvest in life include:

- engaging in an area of interest such as learning a new craft
- enrolling in a class at the university

- volunteering to work for a cause that he believes in
- getting a new job
- learning yoga
- taking a trip

Strategies for discussion that can be employed by the nurse-healer that encourage the griever to reinvest in life include:

- discussion of life changes that occurred because of the death
- exploration of feelings (both positive and negative) of the future
- exploration of feelings associated with forming new relationships
- discussion concerning the positive impact of the death
- discussion of the possibility of personal growth
- exploration of any guilt associated with forming new relationships
- exploration of future goals

Accomplishment of the task of reinvesting in life may occur quietly and slowly. For example, when reinvestment in life occurs slowly, the individual may suddenly discover that a day or two has gone by without thoughts of the lost loved one. A decision is made without turmoil. New relationships and activities are seen as pleasurable rather than something to simply fill the time. The revelation that life is good again may occur spontaneously, although the change has been slowly occurring and has been filled with pitfalls and setbacks. This gradual reinvestment period may be marked with varying degrees of guilt. This period is also the period of empowerment discussed in the earlier section on connecting. As the client feels empowered to manage life again, the time needed with the nurse will decrease. Closure may occur either formally or informally.

In others, the task of reinvestment is one that does not occur slowly, but abruptly. For these individuals, reinvestment in life is a conscious choice. One example is an individual who, after grieving for his wife for over a year, suddenly stated "I have grieved long enough. It is time to move on." From the point of this statement, the individual made a conscious effort to move toward beginning a new life with new relationships and new direction.

This reinvestment in life does not necessarily mean that all problems are solved; rather it brings the realization that the death can be used as a stepping stone for growth. Growth can be exhibited in the following ways: feeling more deeply, empathizing more fully, caring more completely, or developing more sensitivity toward others in similar circumstances. These attributes can make the griever aware of the importance of relationships. When relationships are valued, the groundwork is laid for better relationships with others in the future.

Resolution

The grieving process has been divided, segmented, and discussed using the tasks identified by Worden (1982). In reality, grief is not nearly so neatly packaged. The phases of grief and the individual responses are often intertwined. Individuals may go in and out of the various phases as progress is made. Feelings ebb and flow without regard to stages and phases. Various healing strategies may be employed in any of the phases.

The result, however, is resolution. True resolution results in accepting the death, reinvesting in life, and forming new relationships. Resolution does not mean never thinking of the loved one or not discussing memories. Resolution provides a greater opportunity to feel the love, the joy, and the sweetness of having this individual as a part of the survivor's life. Resolution provides freedom to grow, to change, to become whole again, and to face the challenges of the future with optimism and courage.

Some will never reach a true state of resolution. Lack of true resolution can occur with any death. However, it is more likely to occur when the death is of a traumatic nature, occurs without warning, or if the death involves the loss of a child (Wortman & Silver, 1989).

Grief that Passes Quickly

Many individuals pass through the grieving process with apparent ease and minimal pain. These individuals require limited, if any, assistance. The extent of pain and grief suffered appears proportional to the griever's ability to relinquish the lost love and reinvest in life. If the griever is unable to sever earthly ties with the deceased, the grief experienced with the death of a loved one may be extremely painful. The loss of someone who fulfills many emotional needs is never easy because emotional turmoil exists until new ways to meet those needs are identified. A person can have great love for a friend, a family member, or even a spouse, yet can let go of the relationship and continue with life. For these individuals, the grieving process may move swiftly and with relative ease. The stages of grief may mesh with no identifiable phases. This lack of emotional turmoil may invoke criticism from others. However, if the premise that grief is individualistic in nature is adopted, then even short-lived grief is acceptable and usually normal. These individuals may have had a close relationship, yet may not have been dependent on the deceased for emotional, social, or physical needs. While the love may be great, they reinvest in life and establish new relationships without intense sadness and emotional turmoil. Those with a deep religious faith may use that faith to sustain them during times of loss. A strong faith provides hope of reconciliation with the loved one in the future.

SPECIFIC HEALING STRATEGIES

There are many healing strategies that can be used by the nurse-healer to facilitate the grieving process and help the client move toward resolution. While the strategies are as varied and individualistic as each individual client, some more effective strategies are discussed in the following sections.

Fostering Hope

Fostering hope is an important role for the nurse-healer. Individuals who have a high level of hope have a greater ability to cope (Herth, 1989). Hopelessness offers no incentive to actively grieve or to engage in the grief work. Grief work is necessary to overcome grief. The feeling that "this too will pass" is absent in hopelessness. The client's attention must be refocused from the past to the here and now. Positive aspects of daily life are emphasized. Hope is generated from within and enhanced by a positive view of life. The nurse-healer must guide the client to develop a more positive view of life. Cultivating an appreciation of the seemingly insignificant things in life can foster hope. Learning to appreciate simple occurrences such as a sunrise, rain falling on the rooftops, a child playing in the sand, or the miracle of life is important. An appreciation of seemingly insignificant aspects of life may redirect thoughts toward a more positive view of life and increased hope.

Other suggestions that cultivate a more positive view of life include: writing a poem, meditating, taking a nature walk, helping someone in need, talking to self in positive terms, self-analysis of strengths, or planning for the future. However, cliches such as "Cheer up, things aren't so bad" or "Let's look on the positive side" do not foster hope and should be avoided. Gentle guidance and a positive outlook by the nurse-healer provides the nurturing environment that fosters hope.

Cultivating Avenues of Support

There are three avenues of support for those who are grieving: professional support, social support, and group support. Professional support comes from nurses and other health care professionals. Social support comes from friends and family members. Group support comes from individuals who gather to offer support to each other for a predetermined reason.

The nurse assesses the strength of the relationship the griever has with family and friends. Often family and friends are good sources of support. Relationships that are particularly supportive are encouraged. Supportive relationships can provide encouragement, a means to validate thoughts and feelings, and an avenue to test new ideas and coping strategies.

Most hospice programs have follow-up bereavement care. This care may be one-to-one counseling with the nurse. Care is also provided through support groups that meet regularly. Support groups are excellent sources of help for the griever. The American Cancer Society offers a five-session support group called "Life After Loss." This program consists of planned sessions that include providing information and encouraging dialogue to facilitate grieving. Various coping strategies are explored and assignments are given that provoke thought and exploration of feelings.

Meeting Physical Needs

Areas of focus in the physical realm include nutritional care and adequate exercise. Proper diet and adequate exercise are healing in themselves. Emphasis is placed on eating fresh fruits and vegetables with adequate amounts of high-quality protein such as milk, cheese, lean meat, poultry, beans, and lentils. Exercise such as running, jogging, walking, swimming, or cycling promotes the release of serotonin, which elevates the mood and acts as a relaxant.

Developing Inner Strengths

There are often unrecognized strengths and resources within the griever that have never been explored. Grief offers the opportunity to tap into these resources. A helpful philosophy that can serve as a building block for developing inner strength is the belief that personal growth is often preceded by adversity.

A study by Lund, Redburn, Juretich, and Caserta (1989) suggested that mourners with low self-esteem exhibit more symptoms associated with grief than do those with high self-esteem. Because self-esteem of the mourner may be low, bereavement programs should include strategies to enhance self-esteem. Although Beck's (1979) cognitive behavioral therapy was developed for treatment of depression, it can be used as a technique to build esteem in the mourner. As with the depressed client, the mourner may exhibit illogical thinking about self, the death, and the future. The nurse-healer uses the principles of cognitive therapy in working with the client. Use of these principles allows the client to reframe thinking patterns about the self, the death, and the future. The client is taught to restructure thought content from negative thought patterns to positive thought patterns.

Kavanagh (1990) discussed the use of cognitive therapy as an intervention for grieving clients. According to Kavanagh, clients who experience hopelessness, anger, and guilt are candidates for cognitive therapy. In instances where the survivor feels to blame for the death, the griever is asked to examine the situation realistically. Ways in which the griever can make symbolic restitution are explored. If a conflictual relationship existed, it is dealt with similarly. The griever examines the validity of the emotion and the value of the behavior triggered by the emotion. The griever then rehearses more appropriate thoughts to substitute when these detrimental emotions occur.

Positive internal dialogue or self-talk is one way to restructure thought content. Inner dialogue or self-talk is a powerful influence in the lives of all individuals. The unconscious mind believes what it hears the most. Negative self-talk will produce the negative outcomes predicted by the negative self-talk. Positive self-talk will produce positive outcomes.

The following negative statements used by grievers prohibit personal growth and healing:

"I can't handle this"

"I'll never get over losing . . . "

"I think I'm losing my mind"

"I'm falling apart"

"I can't live without . . . "

"My life is in shambles because . . . "

The unconscious mind believes these statements and behaviors that reinforce the reality of these statements surface.

Using the cognitive behavioral model, the nurse-healer guides the griever in becoming more aware of the words used when talking to the self. The griever is asked to list any negative self-talk and keep a record of such statements. During a session, the nurse-healer helps the griever to rephrase negative statements in a positive framework. For example, "I can't handle this" is rephrased to "I am handling this well." Or the phrase, "I can't live without . . ." is changed to "I wish that it were possible to have . . . with me, but I can be happy and content with my life as it is." Other statements that can be incorporated into internal dialogue to facilitate healing include:

"I feel in total control. My body, mind, and spirit are working together to make me the very best that I can be."

"I can accomplish my goals. I can change this problem into an avenue for growth."

"I look forward to each day. Each day is a new adventure that I can handle with ease and confidence."

To become conscious of negative self-talk and replace negative statements with positive ones takes tremendous effort, but the results are worth the effort. The client can gain power over feelings and guide the grieving process in ways that will result in personal growth and healing. The technique of positive self-talk can empower the individual with a healing strategy to maintain balance and harmony when dealing with any of life's issues.

Inner strength and feelings of control can also be enhanced by increasing the knowledge of the grieving process. The griever needs a knowledge of the grieving process. Understanding the instability of the grieving process and the individualistic nature of grief will allow the client to know what to expect.

Spirituality

Spirituality is defined as "a sense of connectedness with a higher power, God, or an ultimate other" (Burkhardt, 1989). For many, a relationship with a higher power is a tremendous source of comfort during grief. Prayer and meditation may also be a source of strength and should be encouraged.

Spirituality may take one of several forms. An individual may become closer to God, resulting in deeper spirituality. An individual may pull away from God, perhaps blaming God for allowing the death to occur. Or if spirituality has never played a large role in an individual's life, she may be indifferent towards spiritual aspects of healing. In this case, spirituality does not play a significant role in healing.

Simply asking the griever about spiritual needs will give the nurse some insight and give the client an opportunity to verbalize needs.

Bibliotherapy

Literature has been used for many years to gain insight and to overcome problematic areas in individuals' lives. *Bibliotherapy* is the term used to refer to the therapeutic use of literature. The term *bibliotherapy* comes from the Greek words for book and healing. Bibliotherapy can be used to convey new thoughts or bring perspective to an issue (Hobus, 1992). *Interactive bibliotherapy* is defined as "a dialogue between the therapist and a client relative to the literary work to bring about a therapeutic interaction" (Hobus, 1992, p. 324). *Reading bibliotherapy* consists of assigning a reading to be used for healing with no discussion to follow between the client and the health care professional (Cohen, 1989). Both types of bibliotherapy can be used by the nurse-healer as healing strategies when working with clients in the grieving process.

With interactive bibliotherapy, the client is given an assigned or suggested reading that will be discussed at a future meeting date. With reading bibliotherapy, no discussion will take place unless the client wishes to discuss some aspect of the reading. Much literature is available on grief and the grieving process. Before suggesting any readings, the nurse must be thoroughly familiar with the needs of the client and the literature assigned for reading. Readings are never assigned blindly. (See "Suggested Books for Bibliotherapy" at the end of this chapter.)

Journal Writing

The act of keeping a log or a journal is a simple but extremely healing technique to use during the grieving process. Keeping a journal allows an individual to put into words his innermost thoughts without fear of criticism. For those who do not feel comfortable verbalizing thoughts or for those who are unable to adequately articulate feelings, journal writing can be very useful.

On occasion, readings pertinent to the grieving process or some problem the client is experiencing may be assigned. The client is asked to write her thoughts and feelings concerning the reading in the journal (Aleksychik, 1989). Writing thoughts in response to an assigned reading forces the writer to focus on the meaning of the reading.

Journals are the personal property of the writer. In general, journals are not shared with the nurse or anyone else. The client may feel comfortable sharing the journal and may do so if he chooses. The healing effect comes from the process of writing innermost thoughts and feelings, not from an analysis of the specific content of the journal.

The client may be asked to set a specific time aside each day (usually 15 to 30 minutes) for writing in the journal. The client is encouraged to meditate, formulate thoughts, and write. Suggested topics for journal writing include:

- special thoughts of the deceased
- feelings that were never expressed
- happy times shared
- saying good-bye
- ways that grief has helped me grow
- living alone
- positive aspects of the future
- new relationships to cultivate

There are countless topics to suggest for journal writing. Some topics become apparent during a session with the client. At times, no topic will be assigned and the client will choose the content of the journal. When no topic is assigned, the client is encouraged to write thoughts and feelings freely as they occur. Times of anger, sadness, or pain are good times to write in the journal. The client may also write a letter to the deceased or write dialogue between herself and the deceased. The griever may find comfort in writing when difficult moments arise. For example, journal writing may be helpful when the client is awakened in the middle of the night with painful memories.

With resolution, the journal becomes the individual's own chronicle of the grieving process. This chronicle can be shared with others, if desired. Generally, the journal proves to be a record of personal growth, insight, and wisdom gained from the grieving process. Some individuals may include photos in the journal portraying the life of the deceased along with cherished keepsakes or other memorabilia.

Relaxation

Relaxation techniques are important avenues of coping for the griever, particularly in the area of stress reduction. The griever often encounters tremendous stress during the grieving process. The nurse-healer can help the client learn a relaxation technique that can be used as a lifelong coping strategy for all types of stress. Jacobson (1938) developed the technique of progressive muscle relaxation as a strategy to reduce stress and promote relaxation. Progressive muscle relaxation can be accomplished by alternately tensing and relaxing the various muscle groups for 5 to 7 seconds each. The process usually begins with the hands and moves to the upper and lower arms, the forehead, the face, neck, back, abdomen, buttocks, thighs, calves, and finally the feet. A more passive method requires the client to concentrate on relaxing the various muscle groups without tightening the muscles first. Relaxation requires that the client focus on slow, deep diaphragmatic breathing and muscular relaxation. The reader is referred to the works of Bernstein and Borkovec (1973), Snyder (1984), and Scandrett and Uecker (1985) for more detailed explanations of progressive relaxation.

At times, the use of imagery helps to induce relaxation. The body reacts to mental pictures as if they were real. For example, focusing on an image such as a peaceful scene, a melting ice cube, a cloud, a beautiful garden, and so on can enhance the state of relaxation. When imagery is used to reduce stress and promote relaxation, the person focuses on developing images that encourage calmness, serenity, peacefulness, and tranquility. The major focus of relaxation is that of a totally relaxed state of being and the elimination of worry. This relaxed state can be healing in itself or it can be used to prepare the client for imagery.

To use relaxation as an effective healing strategy, consistent times must be set aside each day. The nurse teaches the client a relaxation technique using cues that the client is comfortable with. A tape recording can be made by the nurse for the client to use at home to practice relaxation. The client is instructed to set aside time at least two or three times each day to practice the strategy.

Many scripts are available for use with relaxation. The nurse may want to have several scripts available for use with different clients. A discussion before beginning the sessions will assist the nurse-healer in determining what cues are best suited for an individual client. An example of a script for progressive relaxation can be found in figure 9.1.

Preparation

- Have the client in a quiet atmosphere and in comfortable, loose clothing.
- Tell the client the purpose of the session is to reduce tension and promote relaxation.
- Have the client sit in a chair with hands placed comfortably in the lap and feet flat on the floor. An alternate position is lying supine with legs uncrossed and arms resting on the abdomen or by the side of the body in a comfortable position.
- Instruct the client to take a few minutes and simply breathe deeply and if comfortable to close his eyes.

Induction

The following is an abbreviated script for the nurse to use as a guide to induce relaxation.

I'd like for you to be as comfortable as you possibly can. Take a couple of deep breaths. Inhale deeply. Exhale very slowly and very completely. Focus on your breathing. Again, inhale very deeply and exhale very slowly. Become aware of your ability to relax your muscles. Allow every muscle in your body to be as relaxed as possible, starting with the feet. Allow the feet to become very, very comfortable. Relax the feet completely. As the muscles relax you may notice a tingly sensation in the soles and toes of the feet. This simply indicates that the muscles are relaxing.

Be aware as this sensation of relaxation begins to move upward from the feet to the ankles. This sensation of relaxation flows from the ankles to the calves of the legs. The muscles of the calves release the tension and relax. The calves become very comfortable as the tension is released.

This comfortable, relaxed sensation moves upward from the calves to the upper legs and thighs. These muscles also relax and become very comfortable. Feel the muscles on the sides of the legs, the outside of the legs, the inner legs, and on the top of the legs become very comfortable and relaxed.

The sensation of relaxation moves up toward the buttocks and toward the pelvic area. Occasionally you may feel a muscle twitch. This is just another sign that relaxation is occurring. The tension of the muscles of the buttocks, the pelvic area, and the lower abdomen is released. The internal organs relax and the muscles that surround them feel completely tension free.

The sensation of relaxation moves up the body to the upper abdomen, to the chest, and from the lower back toward the upper back. The muscles are relaxing from the chest and the upper back to the shoulders.

This relaxation extends to the neck and the throat. Feel the tension draining from the back of the neck. Tension is draining away from the back of the neck and the back of the head. As tension drains away a sense of relaxation settles in. These feelings are so comfortable and so pleasant. Feel the muscles of the throat, the jaw, and across the bridge of the nose relaxing.

The tension in the arms is released and these muscles feel relaxed. Relaxation spreads to the hands and the fingers as the tension in these areas is released.

From the feet, to the head, to the arms, to the fingertips, the whole body is completely and totally relaxed. Take a few moments to savor this comfortable state of total relaxation of body and mind.

Closure

- Allow time for the client to appreciate this restful state of complete relaxation.
- After a few minutes instruct the client to bring his attention back to the present. At times the nurse may want to count slowly from one to ten as the client progressively returns to a more wakeful state.

FIGURE 9.1 Eliciting the relaxation response.

Imagery

Imagery and relaxation are complementary strategies. Imagery is a process by which visualization is used to problem solve, reduce stress, or develop a more positive view of life. It is a way to quiet and connect the body and the mind through focused attention. Relaxation is a state of being in which the body and mind are in a state of reduced tension. A state of relaxation prepares the client for imagery.

Imagery is called guided imagery when the nurse serves as a guide for the client to develop an imagery scenario through which healing occurs. Imagery is the use of the mind's eye to imagine or visualize a desired outcome or the accomplishment of a goal. The words *imagery* and *visualization* are often used interchangeably.

According to Dossey et al. (1995), memory is "state-bound." That is, what a person learns and remembers depends on the individual's psychological state at the time of the experience. Emotions experienced when an individual is in a severely stressful or uncomfortable state become imbedded in the memory. Imbedded memories or emotions can surface in the grieving process, particularly if the griever has some unresolved conflict with the deceased. Imagery can help the griever to focus on these problems and reframe experiences in a more positive manner. According to Dossey et al. (1995), reframing allows a person to let go of feelings and thoughts that block healing. Using imagery, the client is able to let go of troubling thoughts, allowing the mind to reorganize a situation or experience in a manner that allows healing.

Before engaging in imagery or relaxation, the nurse and the client must mutually decide upon goals for the session. Possible goals for those who are grieving include:

- reduction of stress and anxiety
- resolution of a conflict with the deceased
- expression of emotions such as anger and guilt
- asking for forgiveness
- saying good-bye

The client must choose relaxation or imagery as a healing strategy. The client is assured that the session is stopped at any point that becomes uncomfortable by simply opening the eyes. The ability to imagine vividly and clearly enhances the outcome of imagery. All senses are used to develop the scenario as realistically and vividly as possible.

The imagery may focus on any issue from a pleasurable experience with the deceased to expressing feelings that were not expressed before the death. The client is told that different images will appear and will come and go throughout the session. The client is encouraged to allow the inner self to reveal ways to correct the problem or to heal. Several sessions may be needed for the griever to develop an image of the desired goal that leads to inner healing.

Figure 9.2 gives a brief overview of imagery. For additional information on imagery, the reader is referred to the works of Dossey et al. (1995) and Achterberg (1985).

When dealing with certain volatile issues, the client may not be totally relaxed. The nurse observes for signs of emotional distress such as facial grimacing, tears, or a change in respirations. After visualization, allow time for discussion about the meaning and the significance of the imagery.

- The client is guided through the relaxation process. See figure 9.1.

- When relaxation is attained the client is asked to visualize a place of peace where he feels relaxed and secure. It may be at the beach with the ocean waves gently rolling over the surf. Or it may be in a beautiful wooded area with a cool, clear stream flowing gently.

- Have the client visualize a nonthreatening setting with the deceased present and visualize the situation or problem to be addressed.

- Guide the client to imagine or visualize a positive resolution to the situation.

- Have the client end the visualization scenario and rest comfortably until ready to open his eyes.

- Discuss the meaning and significance of the imagery with the client to develop insight and healing.

- If the client experiences discomfort during the imagery session, address these feelings. This may allow the client to gain insight or resolve issues, thereby allowing healing to proceed.

FIGURE 9.2   Techniques of imagery.

As the grief process progresses, closure or ending the stage of active grief may become a focus. Closure can be facilitated by visualization of saying good-bye, revealing unspoken messages, or reconciliation. Some sessions may focus on building self-esteem or reinvesting in life. Other sessions focus on stress reduction.

Benefits of Imagery and Relaxation   In working with the bereaved, visualization and relaxation techniques can provide methods of coping that serve as outlets for emotions, help overcome the effects of grief, and reduce anxiety. Imagery or visualization can serve as a much-needed cathartic to pave the way for healing. Regardless of the focus of the specific session, the outcome should be on the creation of inner calmness, tranquility, and healing. Clients who learn the benefits of imagery and relaxation can incorporate these techniques into their lifestyle. These strategies can then be used to maintain equilibrium and balance in every area of life.

SUMMARY

Nurses are in a unique position to provide support and guidance to those coping with grief. However, before nurses can help others, they must look inward at themselves. Self-analysis occurs in the spiritual, emotional, mental, and physical domains. Self-analysis should also occur concerning the relationship between the nurse and others. Self-analysis will help the nurse to identify and develop healing qualities that will enable the nurse to become a participant in the healing process. Nurse-healer characteristics foster a healing environment.

Worden's (1982) four tasks of grief form a framework for successful grieving. The tasks include: accepting the loss, experiencing the pain of the loss, rediscovering meaning in life, and reinvesting in life. Specific healing strategies that can be used in working with individuals who have suffered the loss of a loved one include: fostering hope, cultivating avenues of support, developing inner strengths and spirituality, using literature, journal writing, and using relaxation techniques and imagery. The specific healing strategies to use are chosen by the individual. The nurse serves as a guide to facilitate the healing.

Not everyone needs assistance with grieving. Some individuals pass through the grieving process with relative ease and are able to quickly resolve the issues of the death and to reinvest in life.

REFLECTIONS

1. Do a self-analysis of personal strengths and weaknesses. What strengths and weaknesses does your self-analysis reveal? What areas can you improve upon? In what areas do you serve as a role model?

2. Do you practice relaxation and imagery?

3. List the statements you use for self-talk. Rewrite negative self-talk statements positively.

4. What healing strategies do you use to maintain a balance in your life?

References

Achterberg, J. (1985). *Imagery in Healing.* Boston: Shambhala Publications.

Aleksychik, A. (1989). Bibliotherapy: An effective principal and supplementary method of healing, correcting, and administering relief. *Journal of Poetry Therapy, 3*(1), 19–21.

American Psychiatric Association. (1994). *Diagnostic and statistical manual of mental disorders* (4th ed.). Washington, DC: Author.

Attig, T. (1991). The importance of conceiving grief as an active process. *Death Studies, 15,* 385–393.

Beck, A. (1979). *Cognitive therapy.* New York: New American Library.

Bernstein, D., & Borkovec, T. (1973). Progressive relaxation training: A manual for helping professions. Champaign, IL: Research Press.

Burkhardt, M. A. (1989). Spirituality: An analysis of the concept. *Holistic Nursing Practice, 3*(3), 69–77.

Clayton, G., Murray, J., Horner, S., & Greene, P. (1991), Connecting: A catalyst for caring. *Anthology on Caring, National League for Nursing Publications, 15*(2392), 155–168.

Cohen, L. J. (1989). Reading as a group process phenomenon: A theoretical framework for bibliotherapy. *Journal of Poetry Therapy, 3*(2), 73–83.

Curry, L. C., & Stone, J. G. (1992). Moving on: Recovering from the death of a spouse. *Clinical Nurse Specialist, 6*(4), 180–190.

Dossey, B. M., Keegan, L., Guzzetta, C. E., & Kolkmeier, L. G. (1995). *Holistic nursing: A handbook for practice* (2nd ed.). Gaithersburg, MD: Aspen Publishers, Inc.

Herth, K. A. (1989). The relationship between level of hope and level of coping response and other variables in patients with cancer. *Oncology Nurse Forum, 16*(1) 67–72.

Hobus, R. (1992). Literature: A dimension of nursing therapeutics. In J. F. Miller (Ed.), *Coping with chronic illness* (2nd ed.) (pp. 323–350). Philadelphia: F. A. Davis Co.

Jacobson, E. (1938). *Progressive relaxation.* Chicago: University of Chicago Press.

Kavanagh, D. J. (1990). Towards a cognitive-behavioral intervention for adult grief reactions. *British Journal of Psychiatry, 157,* 373–383.

Lindemann, I. (1944). Symptomatology and management of acute grief. *American Journal of Psychiatry, 101,* 141–148.

Lund, D., Redburn, D., Juretich, M., & Caserta, M. (1989). Resolving problems implementing bereavement self-help groups. In D.A. Lund (Ed.), *Older bereaved spouses: Research with practical applications* (pp. 203–216). New York: Taylor & Francis/Hemisphere.

McIntosh, D. N., Silver, R. C., & Wortman, C. B. (1993). Religion's role in adjustment to a negative life event: Coping with the loss of a child. *Journal of Personality and Social Psychology, 65*(4), 812–821.

Moberg, D. (1979). *Spiritual well-being: Sociological perspectives.* Washington, DC: University Press of America.

Perls, F. (1951). *Gestalt therapy.* New York: Julian Press.

Powell, J. (1969). *Why am I afraid to tell you who I am?* Niles, IL: Argus Communications.

Scandrett, S., & Uecker, S. (1985). Relaxation training. In G. M. Bulechek & J. C. McCloskey (Eds.), *Nursing interventions: Treatments for nursing diagnosis* (pp. 22–48). Philadelphia: Saunders.

Snyder, M. (1984). Progressive relaxation as a nursing intervention: An analysis. *Advances in Nursing Science, 6*(3), 47–58.

Vargas, L. A., Loya, F., & Hodde-Vargas, J. (1989). Exploring the multidimensional aspects of grief reaction. *American Journal of Psychiatry, 146*(11), 1484–1488.

Worden, W. (1982). *Grief counseling and grief therapy.* New York: Springer.

Wortman, C. B., & Silver, R. C. (1989). The myths of coping with loss. *Journal of Consulting and Clinical Psychology, 57*(3), 349–357.

Suggested Books for Bibliotherapy

Akner, L. (1993). *How to survive the loss of a parent: A guide for adults.* New York: William Morrow & Co., Inc.

Arnold, J. H. (1983). *A child dies: Portrait of family grief.* Gaithersburg, MD: Aspen Publishers.

Biebel, D. (1989). *If God is so good, Why do I hurt so bad?* Colorado Springs, CO: NAV Press.

Biebel, D. (1974). *Jonathan you left too soon.* New York: Signet.

Caine, L. (1974). *On being a widow.* New York: William Morrow & Co.

Colgrove, M., Bloomfield, H. H., & McWilliams, P. (1976). *How to survive the loss of a love.* New York: Bantam Books, Inc.

Ericsson, S. (1988). *Companion through the darkness.* New York: Harper Perennial.

Freedman, R. (1995). Overcoming loss: A healing guide. White Plains, NY: Peter Pauper Press, Inc.

Ginsburg, G. D. (1987). *To live again.* Los Angeles, CA: Jeremy P. Tarcher, Inc.

Grollman, E. (1977). *Living when a loved one has died.* Boston: Beacon Press.

Lightner, C., & Hathaway, N. (1990). *Giving sorrow words.* New York: Warner Books, Inc.

Manning, D. (1979). *Don't take my grief away.* New York: Harper & Row.

Sterns, A. K. (1984). *Living through personal crisis.* New York: Ballantine Books.

Tatelbaum, J. (1980). *The courage to grieve.* New York: Harper & Row.

Books for Children

Anderson, L. (1980). *Death.* New York: First Book.

Bradley, B. (1979). *Endings: A book about death.* Reading, MA: Addison-Wesley.

Bunting, E. (1982). *The happy funeral.* New York: Harper & Row.

Buscaglia, L. (1982). *The fall of Freddie the leaf.* Thorofare, NJ: Charles B. Slack.

Clifton, L. (1983). *Everett Anderson's good-bye.* New York: Holt, Rinehart, & Winston.

Cohen, M. (1984). *Jim's dog Muffin.* New York: Greenwillow.

Grollman, E. (1990). *Talking about death: A dialogue.* New York: G. P. Putnam & Sons.

Krementz, J. (1981). *How it feels when a parent dies.* New York: Alfred A. Knopf.

Kübler-Ross, E. (1993). *On children and death.* New York: Simon & Schuster.

Leshan, E. (1976). *Learning to say good-bye.* New York: Macmillan.

Rofes, E. (1985). *The kid's book about death and dying.* Boston: Little Brown.

Simon, N. (1986). *The saddest time.* Niles, IL: Albert Whitmont.

Stein, S. (1974). *About dying: An open book for patients and children together.* New York: Walker & Co.

Viorst, J. (1971). *The tenth good thing about Barney.* Atheneum, NY: Connecticut Printers.

10 GROWING THROUGH GRIEF

Beatriz C. Nieto

> *He will wipe every tear from their eyes, and death shall be no more, neither shall there be mourning nor crying nor pain any more, for the former things have passed away.*

Rev. 21:4, RSV

INTRODUCTION

Throughout the previous chapters, different concepts and theories on death, dying, and bereavement have been introduced. Along with these theories and concepts, stories of people and how their lives have been changed due to suffering a loss, and how they coped, have also been included. This chapter focuses on communicating to the reader how others have grown and learned from going through the most devastating event of their lives; that of losing someone they loved or cared for.

LESSONS OF LIFE

There are many lessons to learn throughout our lifetime. From the moment we are born, our lives are filled with adventures that help us to grow and develop physically, emotionally, psychologically, and spiritually. As children, we depend on our parents or others to provide for and fulfill our needs. We learn to walk and talk and to develop relationships with different individuals. According to Sullivan and Guntzelman (1991), we begin very early in life to define ourselves by all these connections. We incorporate many persons, ideas, and aspects of experience into ourselves.

A child may feel a sense of loss when left at a day care center, a baby-sitter's house, or at school for the first time. He may experience separation anxiety when the parent leaves. This may be the beginning of a lesson in loss and learning to cope with the loss.

As we embark on our teenage years, life's lessons become more complicated, primarily because of the confusion that accompanies this stage of development. Lessons about our sexuality, self-esteem, peer pressure, and experimentation with drugs and alcohol are prevalent during this time. The teenage years are filled with ambivalent feelings and emotions regarding family, love, independence, and making choices between right and wrong. A teenager may feel trapped between no longer being a child and not yet being considered an adult. She may feel a sense of loss for what used to be. It is also not uncommon for a teenager to face the death of a friend due to drugs, motor vehicle accidents, and/or suicide.

Fortunately, our teenage years do not last forever, but with age comes different responsibilities and concerns. Marriage, career, and having children fill the lives of most young adults. In the midst of their busy lives, they may experience the death of a grandparent, an older aunt or uncle, or someone close to the family. They may experience feelings of sadness and grief because the loss may have occurred closer to home and they may be beginning to realize the reality of death. Expressing feelings about death is very difficult because death is a topic nobody really wants to talk about or even think about.

As the future becomes the present, our lives are again filled with different responsibilities and concerns. We are older, our children are grown, and our parents are now elderly. We are once again faced with learning and coping with new lessons in life. Major concerns at this time may be having to care for our aging parents and/or coming to grips with the death of one or both parents. This reality may be the hardest lesson to take, because it makes us realize that we are not immortal and that death is inevitable.

Every stage of growth and development brings with it many opportunities and challenges. Each stage is a wealth of experiences that enables us to connect and/or identify with many things in life. These opportunities, challenges, and experiences tell us something about who we are, what we think, and how we will handle different situations that arise during our lifetime.

LEARNING THROUGH NURSING

Much like life's lessons, nursing provides us with many challenges and adventures of its own. Being a nurse is a demanding profession no matter what area of nursing we choose. As nurses, our main objective is to provide the highest quality patient care possible to promote healing, coping, and, ultimately, wellness. We are faced with life and death situations on a daily basis. Our roles are vast and many, and the role we assume will depend on what the situation calls for at the time.

Although most of our patients manage to regain their health and can continue their everyday lives, there will be times when we are faced with the death of a patient. The death of a patient is never easy. One nurse shares with us her feelings about a patient's death in the following vignette.

Reactions to Death

A loss or death can occur anywhere at anytime. No one is immune to death. The emotions you feel when you share in someone's death are inexplicable. There is nothing you can say or do that will make the situation better or easier. There is a numbness that takes over your body and everything around you seems to be moving in slow motion. You cannot hear a sound, it is like someone covered your

ears and all you can hear is silence. Then you start wondering
whether you are dreaming, that this cannot be real, or that if only
you had done something different, this would not have happened.

Alas, the numbness begins to subside and reality hits you like a
ton of bricks. You hear family members and others crying and talking
and you see someone holding the loved one's hand and whispering
that he loves her. You see some praying quietly, while others just
stare in disbelief. No matter how prepared you think you are, death
is so incomprehensible, so final. One moment the person is breathing
and the next moment he is not. His body lies so still and so quiet.
You search the person's face for signs of life—a blink of an eye, a
sigh, or the twitch of a muscle—but it never comes.

Another nurse writes about the death of her mother and the
double role she played, that of daughter and nurse. She brings
to light the many lessons that she learned from this very special
patient.

Losing Someone You Love

The most challenging job I have ever had was caring for my mother
during the last few months of her life. Little did I know that all my
preparation as a nurse would be utilized to care for someone that I
cared for and loved so much. The tremendous courage she had till
the very end will always be engraved in my mind. Never had I had
the opportunity to share with someone the intimate act of dying. I
say intimate because we were able to share our faith, beliefs, hopes,
dreams, and even our disappointments.

The fact that I was a nurse gave me the means to handle the
difficult tasks and situations that occurred as her health declined day
by day. This was true because as a nurse I knew I could be profes-

sional and organize her care. I was available to provide her with the help and support she needed. I thought it helped me to better handle the situation.

As her body deteriorated before my eyes, the reality of losing her began to weigh heavily in my heart. It got harder and harder to distinguish between my roles. What made it even harder was the fact that all my family seemed to depend on me to know all the answers. What helped at this point were my colleagues who worked with the hospice program in which my mom was a patient. They reminded me that I was her daughter and that I had the right to feel sad and to cry if I needed to do so.

Their comfort and my mom's courage and determination to keep going gave me the fortitude I needed to meet all my obligations, including taking care of all her needs. At times, the situation would get so bad that I would go home with a broken heart, feeling hopeless, helpless, and useless. But in the morning, her loving spirit would elevate me again and would help me make it through one more day.

During the time of her illness, I learned many important lessons. She taught me the importance of establishing a loving and supportive relationship with the people we care for each day. I learned the importance of having faith and never taking life for granted. For when death comes, it is always too soon. She taught me the importance of being honest, to never give up, and to always love and take care of each other.

During the time of her dying, I learned how important it was for her that her family let go and not have regrets. She told all of us that she was ready and it was her time to go. One week after her 74th birthday, she died in my arms surrounded by all her family.

My mom left me with many memories that will always have a special place in my heart. As her only daughter, I feel I was the only one who had the privilege of sharing the many intimate challenges and truths that occurred during the final journey of her life.

This experience has made me realize the importance of listening and being attuned to what patients and family members may tell you, especially those afflicted with a terminal illness. It has made me aware of my own feelings about death and dying. I feel more secure in helping others to learn about the many aspects of this great mystery of life.

Our role as nurse, caregiver, or nurse-healer may not always be well-delineated, especially when dealing with death and dying. There are no easy answers, no written policy or procedure that will give us the steps to take to arrive at the point where we will feel comfortable enough to help our patients and families deal with death and dying. One nurse brings this point to light as she writes about her experience as a novice nurse working with a patient who was not ready to die.

When a Patient Is Not Ready to Die

Although I have dealt with many deaths throughout my 17 years as a clinical nurse, my experience 2 years out of school as a new intensive care nurse has always stayed with me. This is probably because that is when I realized that sometimes people die before they are ready for death.

This patient was a female in her mid-40s, with a failing heart. Probably her only hope for survival would have been a heart transplant. She was admitted to our ICU on my shift. She was in awful physical condition, but her mind was clear and intact. This patient was a fighter. She told the doctor and me to do whatever we had to; just keep her alive. With essentially no blood pressure and a very high fever, I could not understand how she could be so alert and all the while begging us to save her. She kept repeating, "I'm not ready to die." I had never witnessed someone fighting for her life as she did.

Before this patient and ever since her, I've seen most people accepting or ready for death. Either they were old and ready to die or they were terribly ill, injured, or unconscious, with death expected by the family. Not this patient. She demanded and begged for life until her last breath later that night. She never lost consciousness until the moment of her death. There was no comforting her. She just wanted us to work on saving her life. There was no acceptance, no peace. I remember feeling very puzzled by the experience, maybe because I could not help this woman in any way. It was impossible to save her life, but it was also impossible to help prepare her for death. She was not ready to die.

GROWTH THROUGH PERSONAL GRIEF

Throughout our careers, we learn to deal with life-threatening situations and to work with many different individuals who need our special care. When someone is dying, it is often very difficult to know how to help, what to do, and what to say (Callanan & Kelly, 1992). According to Callanan and Kelly (1992), if we as nurses know how to listen and what to look for, the dying themselves can often supply the answers, letting us know what they need to hear and express to allay their fears and face death with serenity.

In order to turn grief into personal growth, we need to come to grips with the reality of death and dying. We need to understand that while death is a very private event, grief is a personal process and recovery can take a lifetime (Adams, Hershatter, & Moritz, 1991). Rando (1984) stated that "in caring for dying and bereaved individuals we are subject to experiences that will demand a grief response of our own" (p. 430). She further stated that "whenever we lose something or someone in whom we have invested ourselves emotionally, we have a need for a

grief response" (p. 430). Worden (1982) pointed out that working with the bereaved touches us personally in at least three
ways:

- It may make us painfully aware of our own losses.

- It may contribute to our own apprehension regarding
  our own potential and feared losses.

- It may arouse existential anxiety in our personal death
  awareness (p. 108).

As nurses, we learn about the grieving process and its many
stages—denial, anger, bargaining, depression, and acceptance. We
often look for evidence or presence of these stages in our
patients and their families, especially those who may be anticipating a loss or who have already suffered a loss.

Though most of us are aware that people who suffer a loss
need to grieve and that the grieving process is individual for each
person, it is sometimes not obvious to us that these stages of the
grieving process also pertain to us. We also have the right to feel
the loss of those we have come to know and care for. As nurses,
we need to realize where we stand in how we feel about death
and dying to be able to learn and grow from our experiences.
Self-awareness is truly a learning experience and not an easy task
to accomplish. Often working with patients who are on an irreversible trajectory toward death is a threat to our senses of power,
mastery, and control (Rando, 1984, p. 432). If nurses do not learn
to cope with their own feelings regarding death and dying and
if they are in situations that call upon them to care for dying
patients regularly, they may soon experience professional
burnout. This, in turn, will make the nurse vulnerable to unresolved personal stress that can ultimately damage the nurse-
patient relationship.

Harper (1977) developed the Schematic Growth and
Development Scale in Coping with Professional Anxieties in
Terminal Illness. This model depicts the process that health care
professionals go through to become more comfortable as they
work with dying patients. The different stages of the model represent the normal sequence of emotional and psychological
progress. Harper stated that growth is reflected as a professional
"gains understanding, knowledge, strength, and works through
conflicts, internal and external, thus adding a new human caring

dimension to his existing capacity to be helpful. In other words, this is the maturing of the health professional" (p. 21).

Harper's model (cited in Rando, 1984) consists of five different stages as follows:

Stage 1. Intellectualization: Knowledge and Anxiety   When initially confronted with situations involving death and dying, caregivers often respond to the situation intellectually. Reactions to the situations may be based on professional knowledge, as well as factual or philosophical issues concerning death and dying. Conversations between the caregiver and the patient are not at a personal level. The caregiver exhibits ineffective means of coping with and dealing with anxiety, which often results in withdrawal from the dying patient and/or the family. Although the caregivers are concerned with the patient and the situation at hand, they feel uncomfortable and are unable to accept death at this point.

Stage 2. Emotional Survival: Trauma   This stage is characterized by feelings of guilt and frustration as caregivers are confronted with the reality of their patients' impending deaths. During this stage, caregivers are confronted with coming to grips with the reality of losing the patient. They also begin to contemplate the reality of their own eventual death. Death, at this point, is dealt with on an emotional level. Feelings of sympathy intertwined with feelings of guilt come into play as caregivers compare their own health with that of their patients. At this point, caregivers realize that the patient's death and suffering are inevitable. They may often feel traumatized as they begin to experience the reality of death. It is not uncommon for feelings of animosity to be prevalent among caregivers as they pass from the first stage to the second stage of the model. Feelings of hostility may occur as caregivers are jolted from the state of intellectualization to a state of emotional involvement.

Stage 3. Depression: Pain, Mourning, Grieving   This stage is considered the "grow or go" stage and is the most crucial of all the stages. This stage involves developing a growing acceptance to the existing reality of death and dying. Caregivers come to the realization that death truly exists and that there is nothing they can do or feel that will make their patient well. Feelings of pain, mourning, and grief are experienced as the caregiver moves toward the acceptance of death and dying. A decision between accepting death and the dying process or leaving the field will be made during this stage of development.

Stage 4. Emotional Arrival: Moderation, Mitigation, Accommodation   During this stage, caregivers feel a sense of freedom from the debilitating effects of the previous stages of the process. They no longer identify with the patient's symptoms, nor are they preoccupied with their own death and dying. Caregivers' emotional responses to their patients and families are appropriate, with a heightened ability to grieve and the resilience to heal from dealing with death and dying.

Stage 5. Deep Compassion: Self-Realization, Self-Awareness, Self-Actualization   This is the last stage of the model and is characterized as the culminating point of all previous growth and development that the caregiver has gone through. At this point, the caregiver can relate compassionately to the dying patient and fully accept the impending death. Because of heightened self-awareness and self-respect, caregivers can provide dignity and respect to the dying patient as well. They have come to the realization and understanding that sometimes living for some patients can be more painful than dying. The caregiver is capable of appropriately assessing and meeting the needs of the dying patients and their families. At this point, the caregiver has grown personally and professionally.

The model, which consists of the five stages, gives us a way to monitor and reflect on our emotional progress as we learn to care for the dying patient. To learn and grow from our experiences, Rando (1984) stated that "we need to achieve a state of realistic acceptance of the impact of death and dying upon patients and families, and an appropriate expectation for our own performance as caregivers" (p. 435).

In the following vignette, a student nurse writes of her experience with death and dying. Her experience is unique in that she was a patient facing her own death. In being so, she was able to bring to light the many emotions and feelings of a patient and nurse facing death and dying.

When One of Your Own Is Dying

I am a student nurse. I am dying. I write this to you who are and will become nurses in the hope that by my sharing my feelings with you, you may someday be better able to help those who share my experience.

I'm out of the hospital now—perhaps for a month, for 6 months, perhaps for a year—but no one likes to talk about such things. In fact, no one likes to talk about much at all. Nursing must be advancing, but I wish it would hurry. We're taught not to be overly cheery now, to omit the "Everything's fine" routine, and we have done pretty well. But now one is left in a lonely, silent void. With the protective "fine, fine" gone, the staff is left with only their own vulnerability and fear. The dying patient is not yet seen as a person and thus cannot be communicated with as such. He is a symbol of what every human fears and what we each know, at least academically, that we too must someday face. What did they say in psychiatric nursing about meeting pathology with pathology to the detriment of both patient and nurse? And there was a lot about knowing one's own feelings before you could help another with his. How true.

But for me, fear is today and dying is now. You slip in and out of my room, give me medications, and check my blood pressure. Is it because I am a student nurse myself or just a human being that I sense your fright? And your fears enhance mine. Why are you afraid? I am the one who is dying!

I know you feel insecure, don't know what to say, don't know what to do. But please believe me, if you care, you can't go wrong. Just admit that you care. That is really for what we search. We may ask for why's and wherefore's, but we don't really expect answers. Don't run away—wait—all I want to know is that there will be someone to hold my hand when I need it. I am afraid. Death may get to be a routine to you, but it is new to me. You may not see me as unique, but I've never died before. To me, once is pretty unique!

If only we could be honest, both admit our fears, touch one another. If you really care, would you lose so much of your valuable professionalism if you even cried with me? Just person to person? Then it might not be so hard to die—in a hospital—with friends close by. ANON. (cited in Enright, 1983).

The need for us to attend to our own emotional responses as we minister to the dying patient is very important. This need was well-articulated in an editorial in *Nursing Outlook* entitled "What Man Shall Live and Not See Death?" (1964). Although the editorial was speaking of nurses specifically, the same issues can apply to all who care for the dying:

> A nurse faces two very grave responsibilities when her patient is dying. She must give life measures—including emotional support—to the patient as long as possible; she must reassure, understand, and, in a sense, share the grief of those who love the patient. Before she can do justice to either, she needs to resolve her own feelings. Her spiritual convictions may need support; her sense of failure must be alleviated; her reservoir of emotional strength should be replenished (p. 23).

SUMMARY

The memories of those we have loved and cared for, who have died, will always remain a part of us. Whether the loss involved a family member, friend, or patient, the experience may, at the least, help us to develop an awareness of death and dying that might not have been there before. We need to nurture ourselves and learn from these experiences. As we learn, we can help others facing a situation dealing with death and dying. We are all vulnerable to feelings and emotions that accompany a loss. As nurses, we too have a right to grieve. Eventually, our personal grief will have an impact on our personal growth.

___

REFLECTIONS

1. Reflect on what you expect of yourself when caring for the dying patient.

2. What constitutes success to you in your work?

3. Think about some of the most difficult aspects of your work with the dying and the bereaved.

4. What are you doing to help yourself cope with these?

References

Adams, J. P., Hershatter, M. J., & Moritz, D. A. (1991, May/June). Accumulated loss phenomenon among hospice caregivers. *The American Journal of Hospice and Palliative Care, 29–37.*

Callanan, M., & Kelly, P. (1992). *Final gifts.* New York: Bantam Books.

Enright, D. J. (1983). *The Oxford book of death.* New York: Oxford University Press.

Harper, B. C. (1977). *Death: The coping mechanism of the health professional.* Greenville, SC: Southeastern University Press.

Rando, T. A. (1984). *Grief, dying, and death: Clinical interventions for caregivers.* Chicago, IL: Research Press Co.

Sullivan, M. F., & Guntzelman, J. (1991). The grieving process in cultural change. *Health Care Supervisor, 10*(2), 28–33.

What man shall live and not see death? (1964, January). *Nursing Outlook,* p. 23.

Worden, J. W. (1982). *Grief counseling and grief therapy: A handbook for the mental health practitioner.* New York: Springer Publishing Co.

INDEX